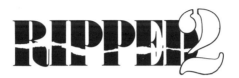

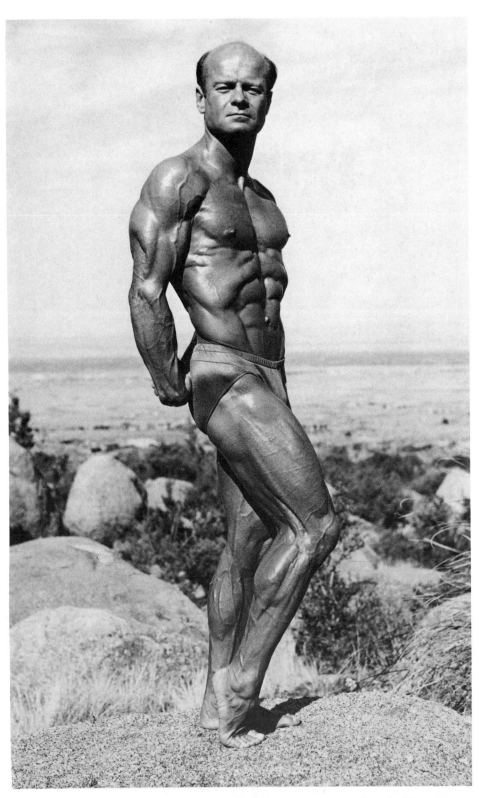

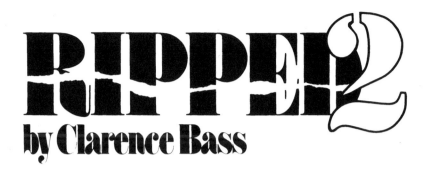

RIPPED 2
by Clarence Bass

The all-new
companion
volume to

RIPPED

*The Sensible
Way to Achieve
Ultimate
Muscularity!*

Clarence Bass' **RIPPED**™ Enterprises
Albuquerque, New Mexico

ISBN–13: 978–0–9609714–1–1
ISBN–10: 0–9609714–1–6

Other Books by Clarence Bass:

RIPPED
The Sensible Way to Achieve Ultimate Muscularity

RIPPED 3
The Recipes, The Routines and The Reasons

THE LEAN ADVANTAGE
Four years of the Ripped Question and Answer Department

THE LEAN ADVANTAGE 2
The Second Four Years

THE LEAN ADVANTAGE 3
Four More Years

LEAN FOR LIFE
The Lifestyle Approach to Leanness

CHALLENGE YOURSELF
Leanness, Fitness & Health At Any Age

Eighth Printing 2006

Copyright © 1982 by Clarence Bass.
All rights reserved.

Published by Clarence Bass' Ripped Enterprises
P.O. Box 51236
Albuquerque, New Mexico 87181–1236 USA

RIPPED™ is the trademark of Clarence and Carol Bass.

Library of Congress Catalog card number: 80–81446
ISBN–13: 978–0–9609714–1–1
ISBN–10: 0–9609714–1–6

Type set by Typography Unlimited
Albuquerque, New Mexico

Printed by Thomson–Shore, Inc.
Dexter, Michigan

Photograph on front cover by Allen Hughes.
Photograph on back cover by Bill Reynolds.

To the inspiring memory of my grandfather, Dr. Clarence R. Bass, who died the year before I was born. He came west from Kentucky in 1903 and made a name for himself in the Moreno Valley gold mining country of northern New Mexico. He referred to himself as "El Viejo Médico" (The Old Doctor) and "The Old Hominy Eater," but he was a strong, gracious man who had a way with words and people.

ACKNOWLEDGMENTS

My thanks to Dr. Michael D. Venters, Dr. Jack A. Loeppky and Lovelace Medical Center for measuring my body composition at regular intervals.

The staff at Typography Unlimited, especially Carolyn Peltier, Janelle Harden and Eric Harden, helped with many of the mechanical aspects of putting this book together, including the art work on the front and back covers. I thank them for doing a fine job.

Bill Reynolds, Editor-In-Chief of *Muscle & Fitness* magazine, took the majority of the photographs which appear in this book. Bill has been a constant source of help and encouragement. I especially thank him for his excellent photography.

Dave Prokop, former Senior Editor of *Muscle & Fitness* magazine, edited my manuscript. He added greatly to its flow and readability. I appreciate and respect his editing skill. Thank you, Dave.

Joe Weider, through his great magazine *Muscle & Fitness*, has publicized my efforts to bodybuilders everywhere. I am deeply grateful for his support and assistance.

Finally a special thanks to my wife, Carol. She helps and supports me in every way possible. I could not have written this book without her.

CONTENTS

FOREWORD

The period following the publication of my book *Ripped* in 1980 was a heady time. I didn't originally plan a book at all. I intended to write a pamphlet about the methods I used to reduce my body fat to 2.4 percent and prepare for the Past-40 Mr. USA and Mr. America contests. I soon realized, however, that a pamphlet wouldn't do justice to the subject. So I decided to write a book.

I began to realize the impact *Ripped* might have on the bodybuilding public when *Muscle & Fitness* Editor-in-Chief Bill Reynolds called from California to tell me he had stayed up most of the night reading my manuscript. He was excited. He said *Ripped* was the best book of its kind he'd ever read. Bill has written several bodybuilding books himself, and he knows bodybuilding. Naturally, I was greatly encouraged.

Bill told Joe Weider, the publisher of *Muscle & Fitness*, about my book. Joe recognized its potential immediately. He asked me to write a question-and-answer column for his magazine. The July 1980 issue of *Muscle & Fitness* carried my first "Ripped" column; it has been a regular feature in the magazine ever since.

Other bodybuilding magazine publishers also liked *Ripped*. Peary Rader recommended my book to the readers of his magazine, *Iron Man*. Dan Lurie put my picture on the cover of his *Muscle Training Illustrated*. Bob Kennedy serialized the book in *Muscle Mag International*. Dave Williams followed suit by serializing it in the British magazine *Bodybuilding Monthly*.

Thanks to the publicity the book received in *Muscle & Fitness* and the other magazines, we got orders for *Ripped* from body-builders everywhere: North and South America, Western Europe, Australia, South Africa, even Russia and places I never heard of—like the Sultanate of Brunei on the northwest coast of Borneo. Men and women everywhere seemed interested in getting ripped. Almost everyone wants to lose fat and gain muscle.

The success of *Ripped* motivated me to further improve and refine my diet and training techniques. Since writing the book I've worked harder than ever to get ripped and stay ripped. I filled five progressively larger training diaries recording my meals, my workouts and my new discoveries. *Ripped 2* is about my post-*Ripped* experiences and the new things I've learned. My first book helped many men and women look and feel better than ever before. I hope *Ripped 2* will help these people, and others, do even better. After all, I learn and improve each year. So can you.

INTRODUCTION: The Principle of Adaptability

Bill Dellinger, track coach at the University of Oregon, teaches what he calls "the principle of adaptability." In a recent issue of *The Runner* magazine, he said, "I think it's a mistake to copy someone else's training program. Each athlete has different needs and abilities. The important thing is the principles of the program."

In *Ripped,* I concentrated on principles and avoided specific exercise routines and, for the most part, specific meal plans. I didn't list my training exercises. Instead, I described the general techniques I use and urged readers to adapt them to their own special circumstances. I wanted readers to focus less on the "how" of my diet and training and more on the "why."

Probably more than any other bodybuilding book, *Ripped* dealt with the trial-and-error process used to find the diet and training system that works best. Readers liked my thought-process approach, but many told me they wanted more detail; they wanted to know exactly what I eat and how I train. In this book I dwell more on the nuts and bolts of my training and diet. I still emphasize principles over specifics, however.

If you're a night person who hates peanut butter, don't despair when you read that I train at 5 a.m. and almost always have a peanut butter sandwich for lunch. Remember, every bodybuilder is conducting an experiment of one. We all have different backgrounds, needs, goals and abilities. Don't blindly copy anyone's training regimen, including mine. I tell you the food I eat and the exercises I use, not as a blueprint for you to follow, but to illustrate the training principles I've adapted to suit my needs.

There's bodybuilding wisdom in the maxim: "Surely the quickest path to disillusionment is the one blazed by someone else." Weigh my advice. If common sense tells you it's good advice, adapt it to *your* special situation.

"The American public has been dieting for 25 years—and has gained five pounds.."

—Covert Bailey, *Fit or Fat?*

PART ONE

Staying Lean

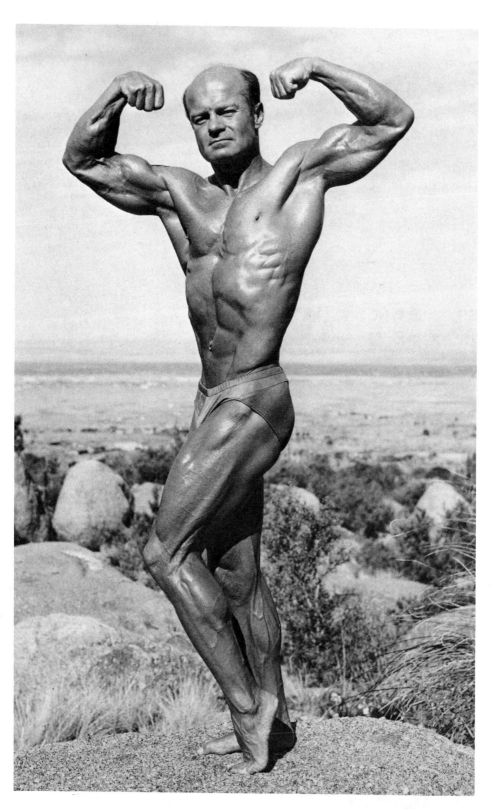

Photo by Allen Hughes.

PART ONE: STAYING LEAN

The Next Step

"The message is loud and clear. Don't try to add muscle by bulking up and reducing down. Become lean and *stay* lean!"

That's how I ended the section of *Ripped* detailing my reduction in 1979 from 9.1 percent body fat to 4.1 percent. To lose nine pounds of fat during that period I was forced to sacrifice five pounds of muscle! That experience convinced me that to make optimum muscle gains I had to stay lean in the first place.

This is a critical point. It's very difficult to lose a large amount of fat without losing some muscle. Exercise, especially weight training, helps to maintain muscle tissue when you're reducing, but, even if you exercise intensely, some muscle almost always comes off with the fat.

Bulking up (the common bodybuilding practice of gaining muscle and fat) and then reducing down is clearly a mistake. Muscle gained while bulking up will probably be lost when you reduce down. The best long-term bodybuilding progress comes when muscle is gained without fat.

Of course, dieting without exercise—a favored approach of so many Americans—usually results in more lost muscle than fat. Many dieters are victims of the "yo-yo" syndrome. They go on a crash diet, lose weight, and then gain it back again. They repeat the process over and over. It's common knowledge that only a small percentage (about one in five) of those who lose weight manage to keep it off. Unfortunately, with each up-and-down cycle more lean tissue is lost.

So on-and-off dieting is a waste of time and energy. The best approach is to lose the body fat and then follow an intelligent diet and exercise program which will ensure that the fat stays off.

I learned my lesson in 1979. In 1978, I had reduced to 2.7 percent body fat. I was careless and, by early 1979, gained 11 pounds of fat. After losing five pounds of precious muscle along with the fat, I was determined to stay lean. I knew this would take some concentration, but it was clear that if I wanted to gain muscle I'd have to keep the fat off.

In the next 29 months, September 1979 to January 1982, my body fat was measured 21 times; it averaged 3.7 percent. That's lean! Top marathon runners, as a group probably the leanest athletes on earth, carry around six percent body fat. Alberto Salazar, the world recordholder in the marathon, is five percent. Derek Clayton, whose record Salazar broke, was measured at seven percent. My low fat levels were 2.4 percent in 1979, 2.7 in 1980 and 2.4 in 1981. My highs were 4.8 in 1980, 5.2 in 1981 and 5.9 in January 1982. Graph One shows my body fat fluctuations over the entire period.

Diet Philosophy

I believe that most diet and nutrition books tend to make weight control either too simple or too complicated. I prefer a practical, commonsense approach to weight control. My method is easy to understand and put into practice.

In a nutshell, my approach is to eat whole, unprocessed foods that are filling and satisfying, but low in calories. Give weight control a high priority in your life, and my method will keep you lean.

Clarence Bass' Body Fat Percentage Compared to Average Males and World-Class Male Marathon Runners

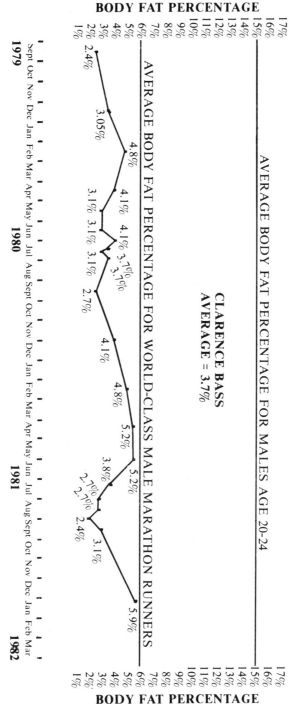

BODY FAT PERCENTAGE

AVERAGE BODY FAT PERCENTAGE FOR MALES AGE 20-24

CLARENCE BASS
AVERAGE = 3.7%

AVERAGE BODY FAT PERCENTAGE FOR WORLD-CLASS MALE MARATHON RUNNERS

17% 16% 15% 14% 13% 12% 11% 10% 9% 8% 7% 6% 5% 4% 3% 2% 1%

2.4%
3.05%
4.8%
4.1% 4.1% 3.7%
3.1% 3.1% 3.1% 3.7%
3.1% 2.7%
4.1%
4.8%
5.2% 5.2%
3.8%
2.7% 2.7%
2.4%
3.1%
5.9%

Sept Oct Nov Dec Jan Feb Mar Apr May Jun Jul Aug Sept Oct Nov Dec Jan Feb Mar Apr May Jun Jul Aug Sept Oct Nov Dec Jan Feb Mar
1979   1980   1981   1982

Graph 1. Body fat fluctuations from September 12, 1979, to January 18, 1982.*

*Body composition tests performed by Lovelace Medical Center, Research Division, Albuquerque, New Mexico.

BODY FAT PERCENTAGE

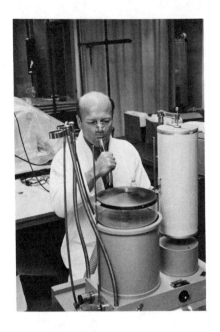
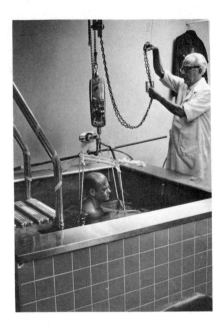
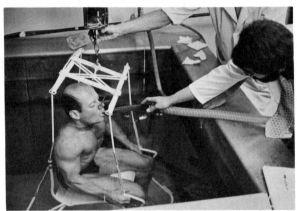
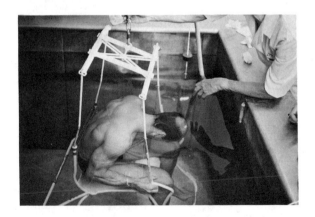

This is one of the 21 body composition tests I had performed at Lovelace Medical Center between September 1979 and January 1982. *Photos by Denie.*

Calorie-Dense Foods Make You Fat

Avoid "calorie-dense" foods: that's the cornerstone of my method. Calorie-dense foods contain a lot of calories per volume. In other words, they provide calories without filling you up. They also encourage you to overeat.

Sugar and butter are the best examples of calorie-dense food. They're high-calorie, low-volume, appetite-stimulating foods. Some other calorie-dense foods are cream, shortening, vegetable oil, candy, ice cream, pastry, jelly and sweetened soft drinks. All of these foods are high in calories and contain little or no bulk.

Most processed foods are calorie-dense. Some examples of calorie-dense, processed foods are potato chips, most ready-to-eat breakfast cereals, salad dressing, catsup, canned soup and most canned fruits and vegetables. In each of these most of the natural bulk has been removed, and sugar or fat has been added. These foods, and processed foods in general, aren't designed to fill you up and make you feel satisfied. They're made to go down easy and make you want more.

Most foods in a box, package, bottle or can are processed. Processed foods are almost always calorie-dense. They stimulate, rather than satisfy, your appetite. They make you overeat, and they make you fat.

Beware of calorie-dense foods!

Fiber Keeps You Lean

I prefer foods that are satisfying and fill me up without giving me too many calories. Foods high in fiber suit my needs best.

High-fiber foods are almost always low in calories. Fiber contains almost no calories. It's the part of plant food that isn't digested. It passes through the digestive tract into the large intestine virtually unchanged. When fiber reaches the large intestine only a minimal number of calories are absorbed through the intestinal wall.

But low calorie content isn't the only advantage. High-fiber foods are bulky and absorb water as they pass through the digestive tract. They fill you up before you get more calories than you need. They make you chew your food, so you eat slower. This gives your appetite control mechanism a chance to signal your brain that you've had enough to eat before you consume too many calories. All the chewing also makes you feel like you've eaten more than you have. As a final bonus, fiber reduces the number of calories you absorb from the other foods you eat.

In short, foods high in fiber help control calorie consumption. The more fiber you eat, the leaner you're likely to be. The best sources of dietary fiber are whole grains, fruits and vegetables. As you might expect, these foods are the backbone of my diet.

Fiber does have some drawbacks, however. If you add too much fiber to your diet too soon it can cause gas. You can reduce this problem by increasing the fiber content of your diet gradually, thus allowing your digestive tract to adjust. Another problem is that a high-fiber diet can interfere with the absorption of nutrients your body needs. For this reason, people who may be poorly nourished shouldn't add fiber to their diet without first consulting their physician.

For more information on the benefits of fiber—fiber is a first-rate cure for constipation and may help people suffering from hemorrhoids, diverticulosis, heart disease or diabetes—I recommend the book *Eat Right* (Arco Publishing, 1979) by Denis Burkitt, M.D.

The Proof Is in the Eating

People often ask me if I eat bread. Bread, along with potatoes, has received a bum rap. Starchy foods are erroneously thought of as fattening. Bread and potatoes are actually good diet foods provided that you eat them without butter. Fruit juices, on the other hand, are usually considered a dieter's delight. That's wrong, too. I eat bread every day and frequently have a baked potato with my dinner, but I almost never drink fruit juice. Some interesting studies support this approach.

In 1975, Dr. Olaf Mickelsen, a professor of nutrition, reported on a study conducted at Michigan State University: "Contrary to what most people think, bread in large amounts is an ideal food in a weight-reducing regimen. Recent work in our laboratory indicates that slightly overweight young men lost weight in a painless and practically effortless manner when they included 12 slices of bread per day in their program. The bread was eaten with their meals. As a result, they became satisfied before they consumed their usual quota of calories. The subjects were admonished to restrict those foods that were concentrated sources of energy [that is, very high in calories]; otherwise, they were free to eat as much as they desired."

Sixteen young men were involved in the eight-week study. Eight were given a high-fiber bread; they lost an average of 19.4 pounds. The other eight were served a low-fiber bread; their average loss was 13.7 pounds. Those eating the high-fiber bread presumably lost more weight because the fiber in the bread made them chew their food and eat slowly. The bread filled their stomachs and satisfied them without giving them too many calories.

In his book *Eat Right,* Dr. Denis Burkett gives the results of a similar experiment in which potatoes were consumed. Twenty-three young Irishmen were fed two pounds of potatoes every day for three months. They were allowed to eat anything else they wanted so long as they ate the potatoes. They also lost weight. Potatoes are bulky and high in fiber. They filled the young men up and kept their calorie consumption down.

An even more interesting experiment was done at the University of Bristol in England. *Jane Brody's Nutrition Book* (W.W. Norton & Co., 1981) provides the details: "Ten healthy people were given test 'meals' of either whole apples, puréed apples (applesauce) or apple juice. Each meal contained the same amount of sugar. It took 17 minutes to eat the apples, six minutes to down the purée and 1½ minutes to drink the juice. It should come as no surprise to learn that the individuals reported greater satisfaction after eating the apples than after drinking the juice, with the purée producing an intermediate level of satiety."

These English experimenters went beyond the subjective feelings of their test subjects. They recorded changes in blood sugar and insulin levels, which showed the physiological basis for the different degrees of hunger satisfaction.

"Blood sugar rose to similar levels after all three meals," Jane Brody explains, "but the insulin level of the blood rose twice as high after the juice than after the whole apple. One to three hours later, the blood sugar levels dropped—back to normal after the apples, but to a level distinctly below normal after the juice. An intermediate but below-normal blood sugar level occurred after the purée."

Brody concludes with a comment on the significance of the different blood sugar and insulin levels in the three groups: "These below-normal levels [of blood sugar], called rebound hypoglycemia, are usually associated with feelings of hunger. Thus, the fiber in the whole apples reduced the demand for insulin and produced a longer lasting feeling of satiety." In other words, whole apples produce long-term hunger satisfaction. Apple juice and applesauce cause low blood sugar; soon after eating them you're hungry again.

So you see, contrary to generally accepted opinion, bread and potatoes are not fattening. And the apple (but not apple juice) is a good appetite control food. My wife always keeps a bowl of apples on our kitchen table. It helps us stay out of the refrigerator.

Say "No" to Low-Carbohydrate Diets

I abandoned the low-carbohydrate, high-protein diet because it made me tired and irritable. I couldn't think or train properly on that diet. As a clincher, I also learned that excess protein is harmful and probably fattening.

Most such diets are high in saturated animal fats (due to the meat and eggs consumed). This can elevate your blood cholesterol level and increase the risk of coronary heart disease. What's more, dietary fat forms a fatty film around your blood cells, causing them to stick together. This clumping restricts circulation in the small blood vessels and capillaries and deprives your brain and other tissues of oxygen. I feel sluggish and sleepy after a high-fat meal. Blood clumping is the reason.

Excessive protein causes a rise in blood uric acid levels, thus posing the risk of gout. My uric acid dropped substantially when I switched to a balanced diet; it was at the upper normal limit and now it's in the bottom half of the normal range. High-protein diets can also cause a loss of calcium and weaken your bones. Further, too much protein makes your kidneys work overtime getting rid of nitrogen wastes.

You need carbohydrates. Your brain must have glucose (blood sugar) to function properly. And carbohydrates are the primary source of glucose. They're also the most efficient source of fuel for your muscles.

Muscles can function on fat and protein, but they don't function well. Dr. Per-Olof Astrand, the famed Swedish exercise physiologist, conducted an experiment which demonstrated this. He worked nine men to exhaustion on a stationary bicycle. On a high-carbohydrate diet the men were able to pedal almost three times as long as they could on a protein/fat diet—two hours and 47 minutes vs. less than one hour! On a normal mixed diet of fats, proteins and carbohydrates, the men pedaled an average of one hour and 54 minutes.

Ironically, a diet high in protein and low in carbohydrates will probably make you fatter than a balanced diet with the same number of calories. Scientists at the University of Virginia fed one group of rats a high-protein diet. A second group of rats was fed a high-carbohydrate diet. The fat and calorie content of the two diets was identical. The rats in the first group (high protein, low carbohydrate) gained much more weight and put on more body fat than did the animals fed meals low in protein and high in carbohydrates. Apparently, on a high-carbohydrate diet, more calories are burned as body heat and fewer are stored as fat.

Fortunately, few people can stay on a high-protein, low-carbohydrate diet for very long. Any weight you lose on such a diet is likely to be temporary. You can't live comfortably on a low-carbohydrate diet. You feel deprived and crave carbohydrates. My advice is: if you haven't tried this diet, don't.

A Balanced Diet Is Best

A balanced diet is the best way to lose fat and stay lean. In 1978 I used a high-protein, low-carbohydrate diet and lost 36 percent fat and 64 percent muscle. In 1979, when I switched to a balanced diet of whole, unprocessed foods, I not only lost weight twice as fast, but compared to 1978, I lost 16 percent more fat and retained 16 percent more muscle. Since 1979 I've used a balanced diet to stay lean.

But what is a well-balanced diet? For some a balanced diet means eating a little of everything. For others it means steak and salad, or protein with every meal, or taking a daily vitamin pill.

To me, a balanced diet must include: 1) Foods from all the basic food groups; 2) The proper carbohydrate/protein/fat ratio; and 3) The proper calorie balance. I pay the most attention to calorie intake, but I certainly don't ignore the other points.

The basic food groups are: 1) The milk group; 2) The meat group (which includes eggs, legumes and nuts); 3) The fruit and vegetable group; and 4) The bread and cereal group. You should eat four or more servings daily from the fruit/vegetable group and the bread/cereal group. Two or more servings a day are recommended from the milk and meat groups. In other words, to eat a balanced diet, two-thirds of your diet should come from grains, fruits and vegetables and the remaining one-third from the milk and meat groups.

In his excellent book *Diet And Nutrition* (Himalayan International Institute, 1978), Dr. Rudolph Ballentine notes that strikingly similar eating habits developed independently in many parts of the world. The pattern that emerges is similar to the North American Basic Four concept—with one significant difference in emphasis. Whole grains, and to a somewhat lesser extent, fresh vegetables, beans and other legumes, make up the bulk of the traditional diets around the world. In these diets, dairy products, meat, fish and fowl are used mainly as seasoning. While the modern American diet relies on an animal-source main dish for protein, the cultures studied by Dr. Ballentine derive their protein from a combination of grain and legumes. I favor the traditional emphasis on grains, legumes and vegetables because these foods are nourishing, filling and low in calories.

The calorie breakdown in both the Basic Four food groups and the traditional diets studied by Ballentine is approximately 60 percent carbohydrate, 20 percent protein and 20 percent fat. This high-carbohydrate, low-protein diet ratio is much healthier than the low-carbohydrate, high-protein diet many bodybuilders prefer. Remember, the brain and the muscles function best on carbohydrate.

Finally, we come to the critical issue of calorie intake. To stay lean you must balance the calories you eat with the calories you expend. But at the same time, you must consume the nutrients your body needs to stay healthy. In other words, you must be careful to get a good nutrient return from the calories you eat.

I want the best return possible for every calorie I consume. In other words, I prefer foods high in nutrients, but low in calories. The best way to be "calorie effective" is to stick with whole, unprocessed foods that have all of the fiber left in and no sugar or fat added.

North Americans favor a "rich man's diet"—a diet high in animal protein and, therefore, high in fat. Fat has more than twice the calories of protein or carbohydrate. The calorie effective way to fill the 20 percent of the diet that should be protein is to reduce your intake of dairy products and meat, and eat more vegetable protein foods such as beans and peas. The protein/calorie ratio of rice and beans is 27 calories for each gram of protein—about the same as steak. The difference is volume. A plateful of rice and beans (1 cup rice, ½ cup beans) contains approximately the same calories and protein as 2.5 ounces of steak, but a plateful of rice and beans is a lot more filling and satisfying than 2.5 ounces of steak.

I try to make every calorie count. I eat foods that are high in nutrition, low in calories and bulky enough to satisfy my hunger. I know I won't get a good return by eating processed foods. They're usually low in fiber and essential nutrients, and high in sugar or fat. In the supermarket my wife and I basically stick to the outside walls where the fruits, vegetables and dairy products are located. The only time we venture over to the inner shelves is when we're looking for dried beans, peas, rice and whole grain items.

You can't beat the calorie-effective, balanced diet. It's the healthiest, most effective and pleasant way to stay lean.

On My Diet It's Hard To Overeat

If you avoid calorie-dense foods and emphasize whole grains, fruits and vegetables, it's hard to eat more calories than your body burns. Eat my way and you can consume huge amounts of food without exceeding your caloric needs. Compare what I normally eat to a typical American diet and you'll understand why. Here's an example of my normal maintenance diet:

MEAL	CALORIES

Early Morning Snack
1 banana 120

Breakfast
Cereal (hot or cold):
  1 cup cooked whole oat groats 132
  1 tablespoon raisins 80
  1 tablespoon Ripped Protein Powder* 34
  3 tablespoons rolled oats 50
  3 tablespoons bran 50
  1 tablespoon wheat germ 26
  1 cup milk** 150
  1 sliced banana 120
        MEAL TOTAL: 642

Alternate Breakfast
1 egg, poached 80
1 slice whole wheat toast 75
Cereal (hot or cold):
  5 tablespoons rolled oats 85
  2 tablespoons wheat germ 52
  1 tablespoon raisins 80
  1 tablespoon Ripped Protein Powder* 34
  1 diced apple (large) 120
  2/3 cup milk** 100
        MEAL TOTAL: 626

Lunch
Peanut butter sandwich
  (whole wheat bread, no sugar, oil or salt
  added to peanuts) 350
1 cup plain yogurt 150
1 raw carrot 42
1 banana 120
        MEAL TOTAL: 662

Mid-Afternoon Snack

2 apples (medium)   200

Dinner

Whole grain rice and beans (1 cup rice, ½ cup beans)   268
1 diced carrot   42
1 diced pear   122
1 cup plain yogurt   150
2 slices whole wheat toast   150

                                   MEAL TOTAL: 732

Evening Snack

Blended liquid mixture:
  1 cup milk**   150
  2 tablespoons Ripped Protein Powder*   67
  1 apple (medium)   100

                                   MEAL TOTAL: 317

                              TOTAL FOR THE DAY: 2673

* *Ripped Protein Powder is my own product. It's available from Ripped Enterprises.*

** *Those who can't digest milk because of lactose intolerance should try adding the enzyme lactase to their milk. A product called Lact-Aid is made for this purpose. Lact-Aid can be purchased at most health food stores and pharmacies, and many supermarkets.*

Soy milk contains no lactose and can be substituted for regular milk.

Now look at a typical American diet:

MEAL	CALORIES

Breakfast

1 cup orange juice	112
3 thin slices bacon	72
2 eggs, fried in butter	200
2 slices white bread with butter and jelly	273
MEAL TOTAL:	657

Lunch

Big Mac	561
French Fries	215
12 oz. Coke	146
MEAL TOTAL:	922

Dinner

4 oz. T-bone steak	536
Baked potato with 1 tablespoon butter	245
½ cup peas	57
Tossed salad with Thousand Island dressing	160
Pumpkin pie	313
MEAL TOTAL:	1311

TOTAL FOR THE DAY: 2890
(Between-meal snacks could easily add another 500 calories)

Note the differences! My diet is made up almost entirely of whole, unprocessed foods. No fried foods are included. No sugar or fat has been added and no fiber removed. The other diet, however, is loaded with calorie-dense foods.

The 217 additional calories in the typical American diet would add up to a substantial weight gain over an entire year. The extra calories consumed would be 365 days times 217 calories, or 79,205. Since one pound of body fat equals 3500 calories, this would result in a gain of about 23 pounds of fat in a year!

The most striking difference between the two diets, however, is

28

in volume. My diet is bulkier and more filling. It requires more chewing, which gives my appetite control mechanism plenty of time to signal my brain when I've met my calorie quota. Unless you simply set out to stuff yourself, it's difficult to overeat on a diet like mine.

I eat basically the same foods each day because keeping my meals uniform allows me to monitor my food intake without constantly counting calories. When I do make changes I try to substitute foods that have approximately the same caloric value.

Sometimes I cut back on the size of my morning cereal and add one or two poached eggs and a piece of toast. I almost never change my lunch except to occasionally reduce the amount of peanut butter. I vary my dinner the most. I frequently replace the rice and beans with a large baked potato. I eat the potato plain, without butter. Sometimes I have a large salad with eggs and toast, or I repeat my breakfast. If I'm short of time, I have my evening snack liquid mixture as a substitute for any meal. It's more filling with a banana instead of an apple. I usually thrown in an egg, too, because I don't want to be so hungry that I overeat at my next meal.

I eat foods that I enjoy. You should, too. There's no need to eat the same foods I do; make whatever changes you want. Adapt my diet to *your* taste buds.

Here are a few more things I sometimes eat:

Whole wheat pancakes topped with fresh fruit.

100% corn pasta shells with fresh tomatoes, cooked and blended with spices.

100% corn tortillas with peanut butter.

fresh green beans.

corn on the cob.

baked sweet potato.

baked acorn squash.

fresh broccoli.

baked eggplant.

watermelon.

cantaloupe.

fresh fruit, all kinds.

lima beans, cooked (not canned).

pinto beans, cooked (not canned).

black-cycd peas, cooked (not canned).

Many acceptable variations on my diet can be found in

vegetarian cookbooks available in most large bookstores. Just remember to *emphasize unprocessed, high-fiber foods and avoid calorie-dense foods.*

It's Better Without Meat

I'm sure you've noticed that there's no meat in my diet, not even fish or chicken. Flesh foods contain little fiber and slow down digestion and elimination. They cause constipation. I'm also inclined to overeat when I have meat.

By skipping meat I place myself in good company. George Bernard Shaw, Ralph Waldo Emerson, Henry David Thoreau, Benjamin Franklin and Albert Schweitzer all avoided meat. Famous athletes Paavo Nurmi, Murray Rose and Bill Walton did likewise. Bill Pearl and Andreas Cahling are probably the best-known vegetarian bodybuilders. Pearl claims he wouldn't eat a steak for a million dollars!

There's good evidence that man wasn't made to eat meat. Our teeth are more like those of herbivores than of flesh eaters. They're better designed for grinding than for cutting. Our digestive tract is also more like that of plant-eating animals. Carnivores have a short, smooth digestive tract so they can digest meat, and get rid of the waste products, fast. Our intestines are long and convoluted, which allows us to digest high-fiber plant foods that take a long time to be broken down and absorbed. But meat decomposes rapidly and our digestive tract keeps the toxic waste products in the body far longer than is the case with carnivores.

I get all the protein I need without eating meat. Bodybuilders gaining muscle need only slightly more than the standard protein requirement of one gram for every kilogram (2.2 lbs.) of bodyweight. Our protein needs can be supplied from vegetable sources. True, vegetable sources of protein are less complete and less efficiently used by the body than animal proteins, but that's not a concern if you drink milk or eat eggs. Eggs or dairy products combine with vegetable proteins in a way that makes them complete. That's why I include milk or yogurt with each of my main meals. The peanut butter and bread combination I have at lunch and the rice and beans combination in my evening meals also provide complete protein.

Of course, a bodybuilder watching his or her calorie consumption has a very practical reason to avoid meat. Bulky vegetable protein foods are more filling than animal protein foods. The four-ounce steak in my example of a typical American diet doesn't give you a good return in fullness and satisfaction for the 536 calories it contains. I limit my egg consumption for the same reason. I get more eating pleasure per calorie from oats or rice and beans than from eggs, and I get less fat and cholesterol as well.

It's simple: you feel better and you can eat more if you don't eat meat.

Daily Checks and Adjustments

To help me stay lean I measure my waist and weigh myself every day before breakfast. I record both numbers in my training diary and note any change from the day before.

I always measure my waist at the same place, belly button level. To keep myself honest I pull the tape around my body before I look down, and I take only one reading. With practice you can become accurate to about a quarter of an inch. My waist measurement almost always mirrors my body weight. Based on my waist measurement, I can usually predict whether my weight is up or down. Recording both my waist measurement and body weight gives me a double check on my bodyfat level.

Experience has taught me that large fluctuations in my waist measurement and weight are usually caused by constipation or water retention. True changes come very gradually, not in inches and pounds but in fractions. To gain one pound of fat you must eat 3500 more calories than you burn, which is unlikely in any one day.

Two days ago I ate chocolate cake and pepperoni pizza at my son's 10th birthday party. Yesterday my son and I finished off the leftover cake and pizza. Today my waistline is a half inch bigger and my weight is up three pounds. I'm not concerned, however, because cake and pizza are low in fiber and cause constipation. Pizza also contains a lot of salt and causes water retention. I know I didn't eat 10,500 *extra* calories (3500 calories times three pounds), so I'm confident the gain is constipation and water weight. I'm now back on my regular diet, and I expect my waist and weight to return to normal in a few days. If they don't, I'll know the birthday party had a real effect on my body fat, and I'll reduce my calorie intake until I'm back to where I was before the party.

I make several simple calorie adjustments when I need to lose fat. I cut back 150 to 200 calories a day by removing the cream from my milk and yogurt (one cup of whole milk contains 150 calories; a cup of skimmed milk contains about 50 calories less). I drop some or all of the bananas from my diet (a banana has 120 calories). If further adjustment is necessary, I reduce the peanut butter in my sandwich.

These minor calorie adjustments work for me and they'll work for you, too. Monitor your condition and adjust your diet on a regular basis; you'll have no trouble balancing the calories you consume with the calories you expend. But remember, your body is probably different than mine. You may burn more calories or fewer calories than I do; therefore, you'll have to eat more or less than I do. Checking yourself daily will provide the feedback you'll need to adjust *my* diet to *your* metabolism and activity level. The main thing is to stay on top of what's happening to your body.

Food Supplements

Bodybuilders and nutrition experts disagree on the need for food supplementation. Mr. Heavy Duty, Mike Mentzer, takes supplements only when he's on a very low calorie diet before a contest. Like Ronald M. Deutsch, author *Realities of Nutrition* (Bull Publishing Co., 1976), Mike believes that supplements are rarely needed by normal people who are on good, varied diets. On the other hand, three-time Mr. Olympia Frank Zane and his wife, Christine, take supplements all the time. When they travel they take along a suitcase full of vitamins and minerals. They agree with Richard Passwater, Ph.D., author of *Supernutrition: The Megavitamin Revolution* (The Dial Press, 1975), who argues that supplements are a necessity in the modern world. Bill Pearl, four-time winner of the Mr. Universe title, is a disciple of Paavo O. Airola, the author of *Are You Confused?* (Health Plus Publishers, 1971), and many other books on health and nutrition. "Food supplements are necessary as a nutritional safeguard against disease," says Dr. Airola. He maintains that "well-chosen food supplements are an easy, inexpensive way to improve your diet and

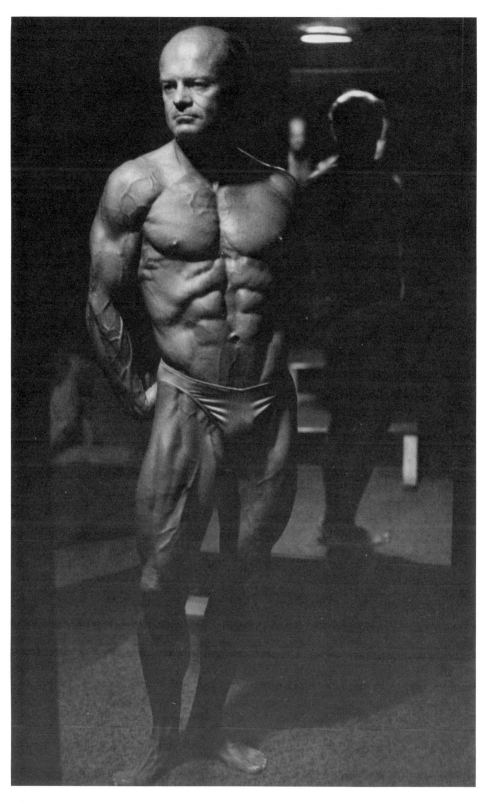

The mirror is an important tool for keeping track of what's happening to your body. *Photo by Bill Reynolds.*

assure optimum health for you and your family."

The supplement dispute isn't limited to bodybuilders. Runners also disagree. The runners' favorite doctor, George Sheehan, won't even talk about supplements. If pushed on the subject of megavitamins and supplements, he usually says, "Whatever turns you on." Conversely, famed miler Marty Liquori, in his *Guide for the Elite Runner* (Playboy Press, 1980), comes down solidly in favor of dietary supplements for athletes in serious training.

Personally, I'm sure that a balanced diet of fresh, natural foods is the best way to avoid nutritional deficiencies. Unfortunately, most of us find it hard to avoid foods which have been robbed of nutrients by processing, storage and shipping. We live stress-filled lives in a polluted environment. Bodybuilders are particularly vulnerable because, like runners, we're always pushing our bodies to do more, and we're usually flirting with dietary deficiencies by restricting our caloric intake.

My father, a medical doctor, gave me vitamin and mineral supplements when I was a child. I've taken such supplements all my life. I make good, wholesome foods the cornerstone of my diet, but I also take supplements as insurance.

I prefer a high-potency, "complete" vitamin and mineral formula which divides the recommended daily dose into several capsules or tablets to be taken with meals throughout the day. In nature vitamins and minerals are found in the food we eat, and they're better absorbed when taken with meals. I divide my multiple vitamin and mineral supplement between breakfast and dinner. In addition, I take a vitamin C-Complex formula to aid tissue repair and protect against infection and pollution, a B-Complex formula to protect against stress and aid in protein, fat and carbohydrate metabolism, and a vitamin E-Complex formula to promote better blood circulation and serve as an anti-oxidant. I also take a chelated mineral formula and a liver concentrate (liver contains so many essential nutrients that it's sometimes called "nature's own multi-vitamin mineral supplement). These additional supplements are taken in the recommended amounts throughout the day with meals.

It's important that you don't try to get extra vitamin C, B, E and minerals by taking several times the recommended dose of a multiple vitamin and mineral formula. If you do, you may take toxic amounts of vitamins A or D. Take the recommended amount of the multiple vitamin and mineral formula; then take extra C, B, and E and minerals separately.

I'm convinced that vitamin and mineral supplements, taken in reasonable amounts, serve as a valuable safeguard against poor eating habits and nutritionally deficient foods.

A final word on protein supplements: bodybuilders only need a little extra protein; in fact, excess protein can be harmful. Nevertheless, on a basically vegetarian diet like mine, a well-balanced protein supplement, taken in reasonable amounts, can be a valuable aid to maintenance, repair and growth of body tissue. I use a protein supplement on my breakfast cereal, especially if I'm not having an egg with breakfast. Also, I often blend a protein supplement in milk with a piece of fruit for a snack or a quick meal substitute. I don't believe in massive protein supplementation, but there are times when protein supplements are useful.

Coping With Calories

Willpower and self-discipline aren't the answer to permanent weight control. You must be comfortable with your diet or you won't stick with it. If you feel deprived, physically or psychologically, you'll fail. You do have to keep in mind the need to balance your caloric intake and your energy expenditure, but you don't have to be in a continual struggle with yourself. I've found a number of ways to cope with calories, year after year.

I try to make sure I never feel hungry or deprived. I eat foods that are filling and satisfying, but not fattening. As already mentioned, I emphasize high-fiber, natural foods. I avoid processed foods that have the fiber and bulk removed and sugar or fat added. I steer clear of foods which give me a lot of calories per volume and encourage me to overeat. In short, I never forget that I can eat all I want of certain foods and still not get fat. Other foods, however, make me fat without filling me up.

By emphasizing whole grains, fruits and vegetables, and avoiding calorie-dense, processed foods, I stay full, satisfied and lean. But other calorie-coping techniques play important supporting roles. I do a number of things to curb my tendency to eat more than I need or really want.

I plan my meals. The only food I put on the table is the food I intend to eat. Leaving serving dishes on the table, boarding-house style, is an invitation to overeat. If you're not careful, you'll be like my favorite comic strip character, Hagar. He "got up too much momentum [at breakfast] and slid right on into lunch."

I'm like anyone else; if extra food is sitting in front of me I'll probably eat it. If, however, I have to get up from the table to get more food, I usually change my mind before I get to the refrigerator. My wife and son help me by clearing their dishes off the table when they finish eating. They know that leftover food on their plate is a temptation I usually can't resist. But if I *really* want more food, I have it so I won't feel deprived. You see, I know that if I feel dissatisfied at the end of a meal, I'm likely to pick between meals or eat too much at the next meal.

I don't leave tempting leftovers around. It's hard to resist food that you see every time you go in the kitchen or open the refrigerator. I freeze leftovers or give them to the dog. It's better to throw food away than to become fat.

The first bite is the most dangerous. If I can avoid that first cookie or the first taste of ice cream, I'm OK. I'm not one of those people who are satisfied with one taste of something. If I take the first bite, I'm apt to eat everything I can lay my hands on. For that reason, if I really want a dessert or some other sweet, I like to have it in a restaurant where it's awkward to have seconds. At home, it's too easy to have seconds, thirds, or worse.

I make sure that I eat slowly. This gives my appetite control mechanism a chance to signal my brain when I've had enough. For example, the raw carrot I usually have with my lunch requires a lot of chewing and makes me feel like I'm eating more than I am. I cut my toast into small pieces because it lasts longer that way. I cut my peanut butter sandwich into six pieces for the same reason. My breakfast cereal and the rice and bean dish that I often have for dinner are satisfying because they're chewy and take a long time to eat. I find that the slower I eat, the less likely I am to overeat.

Backsliding is OK. It takes the pressure off. In fact, an occasional eating splurge is a good idea. If I continually deny myself a trip to Pizza Hut or Baskin-Robbins, I start feeling deprived, and that's a mistake. But if I have my fling occasionally, I'm happy to go back to my regular eating pattern the next day.

The idea is to eat smart. Choose foods that fill you up without making you fat. Don't tempt yourself needlessly. And don't be too strict with yourself. The way to stay the course is to bend a little.

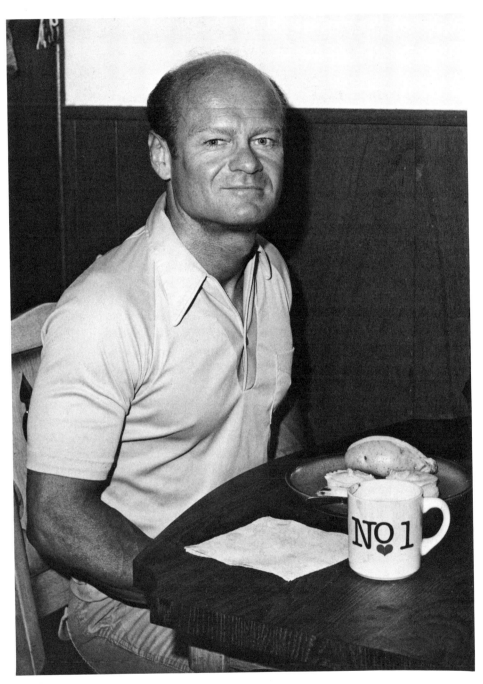

The idea is to eat smart. *Photo by Bill Reynolds.*

These are the calorie-control techniques I've found most helpful. Mark Bricklin's book, *Lose Weight Naturally* (Rodale Press, 1979), has other useful weight-control ideas.

31 Pounds of Fat

I walked off at least 31 pounds of fat last year!

In the fall of 1980 my wife and I started walking two miles each day. By the end of the year we were up to three miles each morning before breakfast. You burn about 100 calories per mile when you walk (or run), so we burned about 300 calories each day. That's not many when you realize there are 3500 calories in one pound of fat. Over the course of a year, however, our three miles adds up to 109,500 calories (365 days times 300) or 31 pounds of fat (109,500 calories divided by 3500). Putting it another way, I'd have gained 31 pounds of fat if I ate the same amount and didn't walk.

If you want to stay lean, it's important that you don't ignore exercise. Increase your physical activity and you'll be able to eat more without getting fat. Walking is a pleasant activity and there are plenty of other easy ways to burn extra calories.

When a parking structure was added to the building where my office is located, I saved money and burned extra calories by continuing to park three blocks away and walking. I almost always walk up the stairs to my office on the third floor. Little things like this add up and they really don't take significantly more time.

You can find many ways to burn extra calories during the day. Take a walk at lunch time or during a coffee break. Stand up when you talk on the telephone. If you want to talk to your neighbors, walk over and see them instead of using the telephone. Don't drive to the corner drugstore, walk or ride a bike.

Use your imagination. If there are two ways to do something, choose the way that burns more calories. Make fat-burning activity part of your daily routine. You'll hardly notice the difference, but your scale sure will.

Increase Your Fat-Burning Capacity

Aerobic exercise should be included in the program of any bodybuilder interested in staying lean. Everybody knows that aerobic exercise burns calories; what isn't so well known is that aerobic exercise increases the capacity of the body to burn fat.

Weight training is anaerobic (without oxygen) exercise. It requires short bursts of high-intensity effort. The energy for this type of stop-and-go exercise comes from glycogen, a carbohydrate, stored in the muscles. Weight training burns almost no fat, because fat can't be converted to energy fat enough. Aerobic (with oxygen) exercise, on the other hand, is low-intensity effort that can be continued for a long period of time. The energy for aerobic exercise comes mainly from fat.

Champion marathon runners like Alberto Salazar, Bill Rodgers and Frank Shorter are veritable fat-burning machines. Long-distance runners "hit the wall' when they use up the glycogen stored in their muscles. So such athletes, in essence, train their bodies to conserve glycogen and burn fat. They do this through aerobic exercise. Aerobic exercise (prolonged continuous exercise) stimulates the production of enzymes that convert fat to energy. The more fat-burning enzymes you have, the better you're able to burn stored fat. In technical terms, aerobic exercise increases your ability to mobilize or metabolize fatty acids. Fatty acids, from your fat deposits or from a recent meal, are carried by the blood to muscle cells. Fat-burning enzymes enable your muscles to use the fatty acids as fuel.

Marathon runners are lean not only because they burn a lot of calories through running, but also because they have developed the capacity to use their body fat as fuel. People who are out of shape, and have few fat-burning enzymes, burn mostly carbohydrates (rather than fat) for fuel. Fit people, on the other hand, burn fat readily. This is true during exercise *and* at rest. The fat-burning benefits of aerobic exercise go on around the clock. If you're aerobically fit, you burn more body fat even when you're sleeping.

In 1977, when my body fat was first measured at 2.4 percent, it was also determined that my aerobic fitness level was 50 percent above average. Putting it another way, my ability to burn body fat was 50 percent above average.

That year my main aerobic activity was a long bicycle ride once a week. At the time I didn't fully understand the importance of aerobic exercise to staying lean. When I learned that aerobic exercise not only burns calories, but also increases the body's fat-burning capacity, I gave aerobic exercise greater emphasis in my

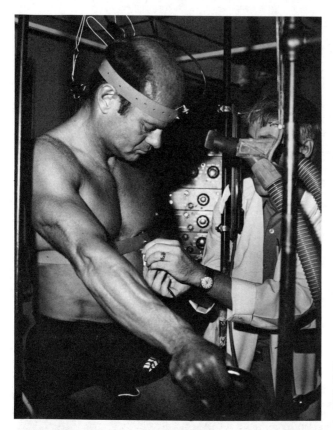

Here I'm getting hooked up for the oxygen uptake capacity test at Lovelace Medical Center. *Photo by Bill Reynolds.*

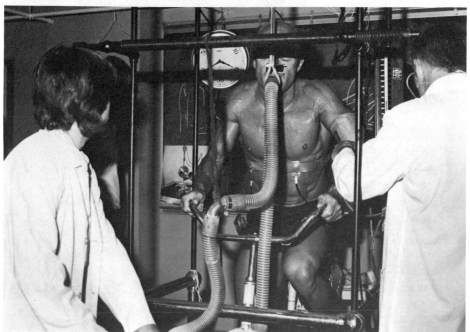

The test is in full swing. A technician collects my exhaled air in big bags. *Photo by Bill Reynolds.*

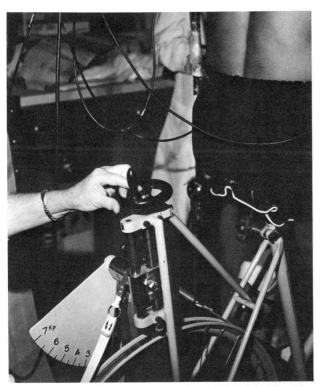

The pedal resistance is increased at regular intervals. *Photo by Bill Reynolds.*

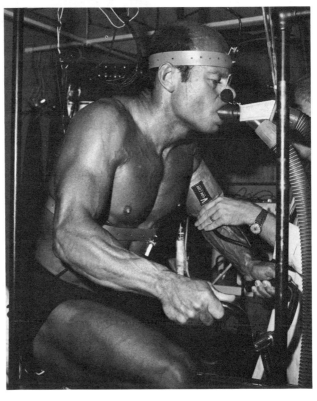

It's getting hard now. *Photo by Bill Reynolds.*

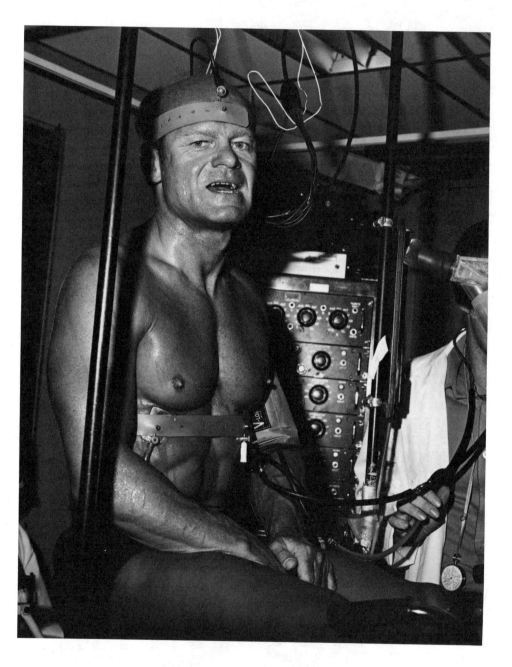

It's over. I hit my limit after 22 minutes. *Photo by Bill Reynolds.*

program. I started walking every day. In the summertime I rode my bicycle every fourth day. Since then I have purchased a stationary bicycle which I ride for 30 minutes most evenings. For variety I occasionally use a rebounder (mini trampoline) and a rowing machine.

Exercise below 80 percent of your maximum heart rate is generally considered to be aerobic. The exercise is anaerobic if the heart rate rises above 80 percent of maximum. Subtract your age from 220 to estimate your maximum heart rate. The average 20-year-old has a maximum heart rate of 200 (220 minus 20) and the average 40-year-old a maximum of 180 (220 minus 40). Heavy weight lifting usually raises your heart beat to near maximum, so it's extremely anaerobic. Walking is extremely aerobic, because it keeps your heart rate well under 80 percent of maximum. It comes as close as anything can to being a pure fat-burning activity.

When I ride my stationary bicycle I usually keep my heart rate under 146, which is 80 percent of my measured maximum. Only occasionally do I push my heart rate higher. I keep my heart rate low to burn fat, but that's not the only reason. I've found I must be careful not to wear myself out with aerobic exercise; otherwise, my weight training suffers. Aerobic exercise is an important adjunct to bodybuilding, but it shouldn't detract from it.

On August 26, 1981, I had my oxygen uptake capacity measured again. I wanted to know how my 1981 cardiovascular fitness compared to my 1977 level. Dr. Jack Leoppky, an Associate Scientist at Lovelace Medical Center, conducted the test. He cautioned me that a three percent loss of aerobic capacity is expected during the four-year time span between the two tests (I was 39 in 1977 and 43 in 1981). But I recorded a better result in 1981 than in 1977—50 ml/min/kg compared to 49 ml/min/kg. My 1981 aerobic capacity was 55 percent better than the predicted level for my age bracket. Clearly, my aerobic exercise program is paying off. My fat-burning enzymes are fighting Father Time, and they're winning.

For further reading on the important role aerobic exercise plays in staying lean, I recommend Covert Bailey's informative book, *Fit or Fat?* (Houghton Mifflin Co., 1978).

Exercise and Appetite

The 30 minutes I spend on my stationary bicycle most evenings before dinner does more than burn calories and stimulate the production of fat-burning enzymes. It helps me control my appetite. Many people, myself included, eat when they're tired, tense, anxious or depressed—every reason except the right one to eat: because you're biologically hungry. I'm not sure why, maybe it's the "high" runners talk about, but the world seems better after my stationary bike session. It is known that the level of endorphins, natural morphine-like compounds in the body, rises during exercise. I think biking also stabilizes my blood sugar level, which tends to be down in the late afternoon. Whatever the reasons, my urge to eat for all the wrong reasons goes away, and I can sit down and enjoy my meal without overeating.

Many people assume that exercise stimulates the appetite. Not necessarily so. Drs. Katch and McArdle, in their book *Nutrition, Weight Control and Exercise* (Houghton Mifflin Co., 1977), explain that we should distinguish between the type and duration of exercise. People who perform hard physical labor or exercise for hours on end do eat more, because their calorie expenditure is extremely high. But vigorous exercise of relatively short duration doesn't stimulate appetite and cause increased food intake.

Katch and McArdle cite a study involving obese young men who participated in a physical conditioning program. Their calorie intake was measured before, during and after an 18-week period in which they exercised one hour each day for eight weeks, laid off for five weeks, and then resumed exercise for five more weeks. Their caloric intake didn't increase significantly during the periods they were exercising. As a group, however, they lost an average of 12.3 percent in body weight. In other words, exercise caused them to burn more calories, not eat more.

Interestingly, there's evidence that exercise has a greater appetite-normalizing effect on fit people than on out-of-shape people. During exercise, the out-of-shape person burns mostly glucose (blood sugar) because he or she lacks fat-burning enzymes. This lowers the blood sugar of the unfit person and stimulates hunger. Exercise has a different effect on the well-conditioned person. Fit people are able to burn stored fat during exercise, so their blood sugar remains more uniform and they don't get hungry.

I can report from personal experience that mild exercise before meals clears the head and puts you in touch with your true need for food. It really works. Try it.

The Lean Advantage

I got a good start in life on staying lean. I wasn't a fat baby or a fat teenager. That's important because fat cells increase in number during three critical stages of life—the last three months before we're born, the first year after we're born and, finally, during the adolescent growth spurt. Once adulthood is achieved, fat cells don't increase in number. They can only increase in size. Studies with rats show that animals that develop fewer fat cells early in life accumulate less fat later in life. The evidence is strong, according to Drs. Katch and McArdle, that "early *prevention* of obesity through exercise and diet, rather than *correction* of existing obesity, may be the most effective way to curb the grossly overfat condition so common in adults." In other words, fat babies and teenagers are predisposed to becoming fat adults. These people have a harder time becoming lean. Still, there's a bright side: when you become lean and fit, it's easier to stay lean.

As already discussed, aerobic exercise increases the capacity to burn fat and curbs the appetite. It's common knowledge that marathon runners who continue to run simply don't get fat. Well-conditioned bodybuilders also have a greatly enhanced ability to stay lean.

Bodybuilders who reduce their body fat and increase their muscle mass find it easier to stay lean. The reason is simple: muscle cells are active cells. They maintain a slight continuous contraction (muscle tone) even while at rest or during sleep. They burn calories 24 hours a day. Fat cells, on the other hand, are inactive. They burn very few calories.

Most of the food you eat is burned by your muscles. Even if you're sedentary, 90 percent of the calories burned in your body are burned by the muscles. Your muscles, of course, burn more calories during exercise, but they continue to burn calories even when you're asleep.

The more muscle you have the more calories you burn. A person with three percent body fat burns more calories per pound of body weight than a person with 25 percent body fat. So a meal that would make the person with 25 percent fat fatter may actually make the person with three percent fat, and more calorie-burning muscle tissue, leaner. In effect, the person with three percent fat speeds along on a high-powered racing engine, burning fuel like mad, while the person with 25 percent fat plods along on an underpowered economy engine.

Bodybuilders who are fit and well-muscled really have a double-barreled advantage. They have extra fat-burning enzymes *and* extra muscle mass to help them stay lean.

The other side of the coin is the person who goes on a crash diet and doesn't exercise. That person compounds his or her problem. Severe dieting without exercise causes a loss of muscle tissue. It also destroys fat-burning enzymes. Loss of muscle and fat-burning enzymes slows the metabolism. Consequently, when the non-exercising dieter starts eating again, fat is gained even faster than before. Such people often gain more weight than they lost. They're in trouble because they've diminished their ability to burn fat and stay lean.

The moral is clear. Become lean through sensible diet, aerobic exercise and weight training, and you'll find it easier to stay lean. Get the lean advantage.

A Training Diary Is Worth the Trouble

Almost everything that you've been reading here was first recorded, in one form or another, in my training diary. My training diary helps me determine what I'm doing right, and just as important, it highlights my mistakes. It charts my progress and makes me think.

I record everything in my diary that bears on my training, from everyday details to thoughts on bodybuilding theory and philosophy. I keep a daily record of my body weight and waistline fluctuations. If I'm stiff, sore, tired or have a pain when I get up in the morning, I note it along with my thoughts on why I feel that way. If I have a cold or some other problem I write that down, too. I sometimes record my pulse when I first wake up, because it's a good indication of recovery. An elevated waking heart rate usually means you haven't recuperated from the training of the last few days. My diary reminds me to continually assess my physical (and mental) ups and downs and how they relate to my training.

I write down what I eat each day. My meal record helps me to adjust my calorie intake to fit my energy expenditure. I record my workouts. I include exercises, sets, repetitions, poundages and the

46

length of the session. I indicate with an arrow whether I should do more, less or the same next workout. I briefly evaluate each workout. How did it go? Was my muscle response good? Did I feel tired? Did I try something new and, if so, is it worth repeating? During or soon after a workout I often think of something I would like to try in a future session. I write it down so I won't forget. I also record my other training activities: walking, biking, suntanning, etc.

I write down my goals and how I plan to achieve them. If I succeed, I have a record for future reference. If I miss, I can review my diary to determine what I did wrong. My diary helps me to avoid past errors and build on successes.

A training diary is excellent for recording ideas. If I read or experience something that suggests a better way to diet or train, I note it in my diary. It's like keeping a pad and pencil by your bedside to write down something important that pops into your mind during the night, or using a napkin to jot down a thought that occurs to you when you're in a restaurant. My diary serves as a place to write down thoughts and ideas for future use.

My years as a lawyer have taught me the value of writing things down. A detailed record facilitates review, analysis and learning. A thoughtful training diary is one of the best guarantees of continued progress. English philosopher Francis Bacon said, "Histories make men wise." A training diary helps a bodybuilder learn from the past and plan for the future.

If you don't have a training diary I urge you to start one. Your diary doesn't have to take any special form. Keep it in the way that suits you best. Why not start today?

Is It Healthy to be Extremely Lean?

It's extremely unlikely that you'll reduce your body fat so low that it's harmful to your health, but it is possible. In fact, Dr. Thomas J. Bassler, a prominent runner-pathologist who studies the things that kill people, says the day you use up all your body fat is the day you die. He says that's what happened to the Catholic prisoners who starved themselves to death in Belfast, Ireland. "There's a study that calculates," Bassler explained recently in *The Runner* magazine, "that the average, lean, fit young man will die after 60 days of fasting." Let's face it, bodybuilders are a determined

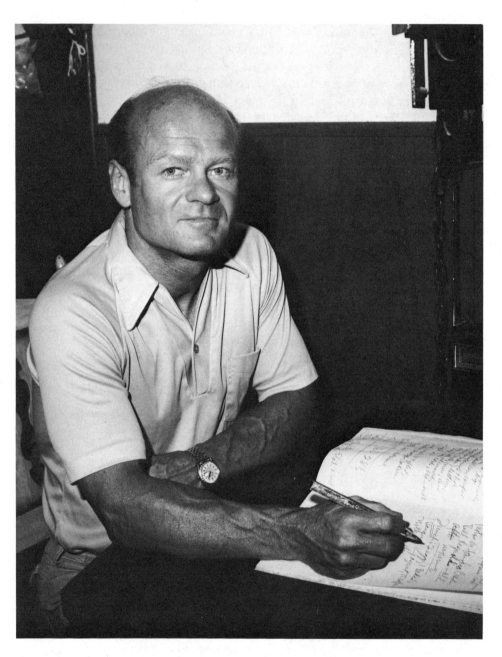

A training diary helps a bodybuilder learn from the past and plan for the future. *Photo by Bill Reynolds.*

bunch, but I don't think very many are that determined.

Body compositions experts Dr. Frank I. Katch and Dr. William B. McArdle tell us that a man cannot reduce his body fat much below three percent without impairing normal function and capacity for exercise. This three percent "essential fat" is the fat stored in the marrow of bones and in organs like the heart, lungs, liver, spleen, kidneys, intestines and tissues of the spinal cord and brain. The body will fight to protect its essential fat stores. Even during prolonged periods of starvation, the fat level in men rarely drops much below three percent.

Many champion male athletes have low bodyfat levels. World-class male marathon runners range from four to eight percent body fat. Drs. Katch and McArdle measured the body composition of the New York Jets football team and found that one former three-time All-American had 3.1 percent body fat, and that two other players had four percent fat. Katch and McArdle believe the low body fat of many champion athletes, especially distance runners, reflects, in part, "a positive adaption" to prolonged, severe training. Very low body fat makes their cooling system work better and reduces the excess weight they must carry around.

Frank Shorter, the 1972 Olympic marathon champion and second-place finisher in 1976, was measured at two percent body fat. He weighed 135 pounds, so he was carrying about three pounds of fat on his body. One pound of fat contains 3500 calories, so his three pounds of fat contained 10,500 calories. Shorter expends about 100 calories per mile in the marathon, or 2600 calories over the full 26 miles. Even if Shorter could get his energy purely from fat, an impossibility, he'd use only three-quarters of a pound of fat in the marathon. According to Covert Bailey, author of *Fit or Fat?*, Shorter actually burns about 50 percent fat, or about one-third of a pound of fat in the course of a marathon. From an energy standpoint, Shorter's low body fat did not appear to be a problem.

In my case, I've reduced my body fat below three percent every year since 1977. Except for a few months in 1979, my body fat has remained below six percent for the last five years. I've had no problems. In fact, I'm more energetic when I'm extremely lean. I walk faster and am more active. I don't require as much sleep. My resting heart rate is lower, in the low 50s, indicating that my body operates more efficiently when I'm lean. Simply put, I function best when I'm extremely lean.

The average man, at age 20-24, has 15 percent body fat. Women of the same age average 27 percent. Men in my age bracket, 40-48, average 22 percent body fat. It's important to realize that these figures are average values. They don't represent desirable or ideal levels, according to Drs. Katch and McArdle.

The extra fat that we carry on our bodies above and beyond our essential fat is called "storage fat." This is the fat—on the abdomen, hips, thighs, and under the skin—that most of us want to lose. In prehistoric times when food was scarce, storage fat was important to survival. When food was plentiful our ancestors ate more than their energy expenditure required and added fat to their bodies. When food was in short supply they used their stored body fat for fuel. Storage fat was a necessity. Fat cells filled up in good times and were emptied in hard times.

In modern times our cupboards are seldom bare. Long periods without food are exceedingly rare. Nevertheless, the average 154-pound man today carries around 18.5 pounds of storage fat. That's about 65,000 calories of stored fuel, enough to live on for a month. We just don't need all that fat. Modern man can function very well with empty storage fat cells. After all, Frank Shorter needed only a small fraction of his two percent body fat to win the Olympic Marathon.

Moreover, studies by Dr. Roy Walford, a pathologist and expert on aging at the UCLA School of Medicine, suggest that eating less may be the key to longer life. Animal studies by Dr. Walford and others indicate that a diet containing all the required nutrients, but about a third fewer calories than needed to maintain "normal body weight," can add the equivalent of 40 years to a mammal's life. Comparable research has not been done on humans, but Dr. Walford believes the finding is applicable to people. "It works in every animal species thus far studied," he says.

It's important to understand, however, that Dr. Walford doesn't advocate malnutrition as a means of extending life. It's healthy to be lean only if healthy means are used to become lean. If you follow an unhealthy diet to become lean, you'll probably be unhealthy.

Some bodybuilders use unhealthy, unbalanced diets to get into contest shape. They cut their carbohydrate intake to practically zero, they adopt extremely low fat diets, they try to live on protein alone, or they simply starve themselves. The body can't function properly on such extreme diets. What's more, such diets are not even the best way to achieve ultimate muscularity.

A bodybuilder who uses unhealthy means to get into contest shape presents a false picture onstage, a mirage. I'm convinced, however, based on my research and personal experience, that extreme leanness achieved through sensible diet and exercise looks *and is* healthy.

How Lean Can Women Become?

A good question. It's generally thought that the essential fat level for women is higher than for men—10-12 percent vs. three percent for men. Their larger quantity of essential fat is found in the breasts and other organ tissues of the body. It's assumed that the additional essential fat possessed by women is related to childbearing and hormonal functions. Drs. Katch and McArdle report that it's generally believed that "the leanest women cannot reduce their essential fat below about 10 to 12 percent." They say, "This probably represents the lower limit of fatness for women in good health."

Women athletes are challenging this theoretical limit on female leanness, however. Body Accounting, a fitness testing facility based in Irvine, Calif., measured the body composition of several of the top competitors in the 1980 American Women's Bodybuilding Championships. Claudia Wilbourn and Kay Baxter, the second- and third-place finishers, had 11.2 and 11.8 bodyfat percentages respectively—right at the theoretical limit. The winner, Laura Combes, was a surprise, however. Her body fat was 7.1 percent! Laura was more than one-third leaner than the other two women. Is Laura one of a kind, an anomaly of nature? Apparently not. Prior to the contest Body Accounting measured the body fat of Susie Green, another top female bodybuilder. Her result was a phenomenally low 5.6 percent! Female athletes are proving that they can reduce their body fat below 10 to 12 percent. But the question is whether such low fat levels are harmful to their health.

Women athletes with body fat below 10-12 percent often have menstrual irregularity. Some don't have periods for months or years. Fortunately, absence of periods (amenorrhea) as a result of exercise and low body fat isn't permanent and doesn't appear to be harmful. In 1979, the American College of Sportsmedicine issued the following Opinion Statement: "Disruption of the menstrual cycle is a common problem for female athletes. While it is important to recognize this problem and discover its etiology, no evidence exists to indicate that this is harmful to the female reproductive system."

Dr. Ken Foreman, coach of the 1980 United States women's Olympic track team, is an exercise physiologist who has studied amenorrhea in female athletes for more than 10 years. He told me, "There isn't one shred of evidence that amenorrhea in female athletes causes premature menopause."

Joan Ullyot, M.D., a world-class marathoner, specializes in sportsmedicine and physical-fitness counseling. She's a leading expert on the problems encountered by women runners. In her book *Running Free* (G.P. Putnam's Sons, 1980), she reports that amenorrhea is common among women runners who reduce their body fat to 12 percent or less. These women, she says, are usually extremely fit and healthy. Dr. Ullyot has a theory that regular, monthly menstruation may be "a relatively modern (10,000 years) physiological aberration which can only flourish in a settled and inactive society." She speculates that it may be natural for very active, healthy women to have irregular or absent periods. Her advice to women athletes with amenorrhea is: "don't worry about it." Dr. Ullyot adds, however, that women athletes who want to become pregnant may find it necessary to cut down on their exercise and increase their fat percentage. (*Warning:* Dr. Ullyot knows of several women runners who became pregnant without having a period.)

It appears, therefore, that women can become almost as lean as men without harming themselves. The caution to women is the same as to men: avoid extreme calorie or carbohydrate deprivation. For men and women alike, sensible diet and exercise is the way to healthy leanness.

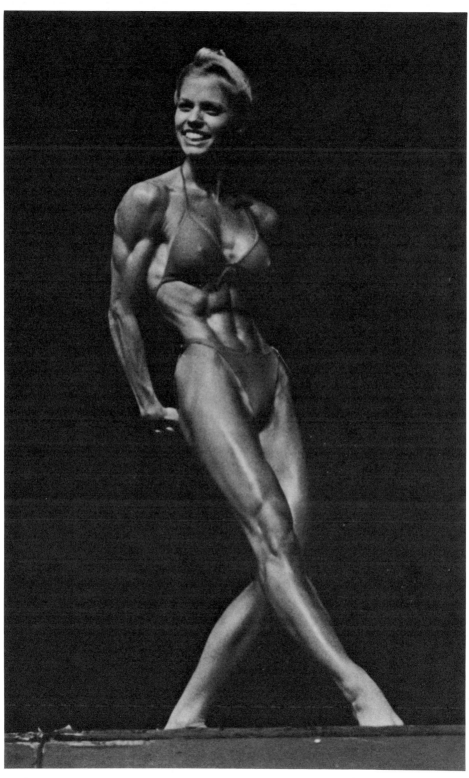

Susie Green's body fat has been measured at a phenomenally low 5.6 percent! *Photo courtesy of Susie Green.*

"[The body] is like a spring—you press and it jumps. You press more and it jumps more. But [training] must be limited so as not to damage the spring."

—Emil Zatopek,
1952 Olympic champion,
5000 meters, 10,000 meters and marathon.

PART TWO

Building Muscle

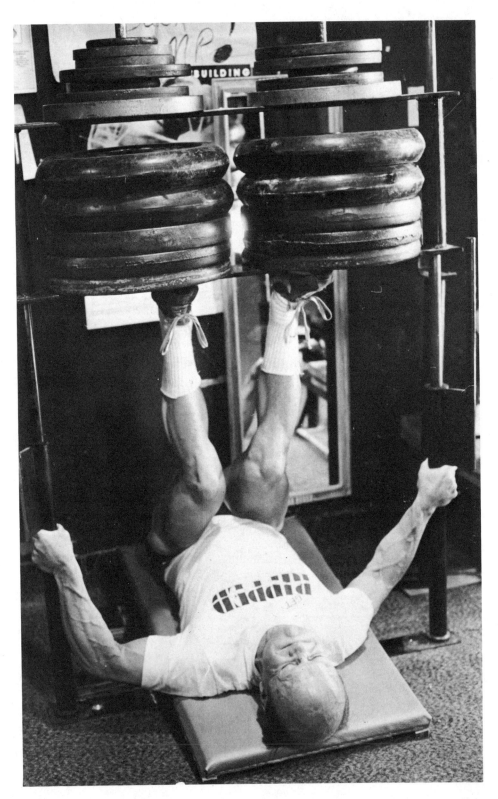

Photo by Denie.

PART TWO: BUILDING MUSCLE

It's A Struggle

"I look forward eagerly to the future when I'll spend my time adding muscle, not taking off fat." On that expectant note, I ended my first book, *Ripped.* In the two-year period, 1977 to 1979, covered in *Ripped,* I increased my lean body weight by a little more than three pounds. My August 24, 1977 body composition test—the first of 16 reported in *Ripped*—showed my gross body weight to be 155.74 pounds, made up of 3.73 pounds of fat (2.4%) and 152.02 pounds of lean body weight. On September 12, 1979—the last test reported in *Ripped*—my fat weight was essentially the same, 3.75 pounds, but my total weight and my lean weight had increased by 3.3 pounds, to 159.09 and 155.3 pounds respectively. A muscle gain of more than three pounds isn't bad for a 41-year-old bodybuilder, but I wasn't satisfied.

The results of my efforts to add muscle during the period covered by *Ripped* and since then are shown in graph 2. In the two years following *Ripped,* I pushed my lean body mass to a high of 163.1 pounds (on August 3, 1981), a gain of 7.8 pounds. That brought my total muscle gains since 1977 to 11.08 pounds. During the same four-year period I increased my leg press poundage by 300 pounds, going from 15 repetitions with 450 to 14 with 750.

My results have been good, but as the ups and downs on the graph show, building muscle isn't always smooth sailing. As a matter of fact, it's usually a slow, difficult process. There are numerous peaks, valleys and plateaus. Nevertheless, getting the job done is incredibly rewarding and satisfying. It's hard, but it's worth it. The thing to remember, especially when things aren't going well, is that the general year-to-year trend is the important factor. If the trend is up, you're doing OK.

All Or None

Muscles get bigger and stronger when they're forced to do more than they've done before. This is the "overload principle" and it's the basis of all weight training. The overload principle works in conjunction with the "progressive resistance principle." As overload makes the muscles stronger, the poundages are gradually increased. Gradually and progressively, the muscles are subjected to heavier and heavier resistance. Overload, progressively applied, makes the muscles get bigger and stronger. Weight training is a continuous cycle of overloading the muscles, allowing them to respond by getting bigger and stronger, and then overloading them again.

It helps to understand a little about how muscle fibers function. When I was a teenager and had been training for only a short time, my father told me about the "all-or-none" law of muscle fiber contraction. When a muscle fiber is stimulated by a nerve impulse, it contracts completely or not at all. A muscle fiber is either completely "on" or completely "off." There's no such thing as a halfhearted or halfway contraction. Muscle fibers work as hard as possible—or not at all.

Even though I was exposed to this law more than 20 years ago, it was only recently that I came to appreciate how important it is to the muscle-building process. Let's see how it works in actual practice.

The body uses muscle fibers sparingly. It always enlists the minimum number of fibers necessary for the task at hand. When you raise a glass of water to your lips, for instance, the only muscle fibers that contract are those needed to lift the water glass. The rest of the fibers in your biceps don't contract. They're held in reserve.

58

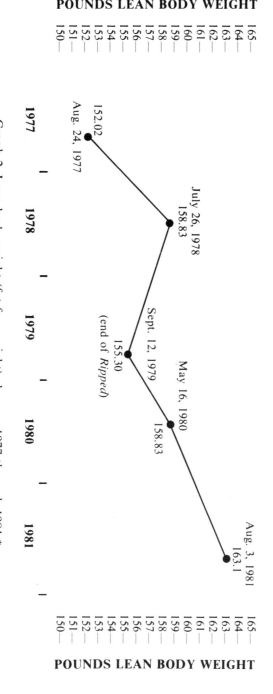

Yearly Lean Body Weight (Fat Free) Highs 1977 to 1981
Total Gain = 11.08 Pounds

POUNDS LEAN BODY WEIGHT

1977	1978	1979	1980	1981

Aug. 24, 1977
152.02

July 26, 1978
158.83

Sept. 12, 1979
155.30
(end of *Ripped*)

May 16, 1980
158.83

Aug. 3, 1981
163.1

POUNDS LEAN BODY WEIGHT

Graph 2. Lean body weight (fat free weight) changes 1977 through 1981.*

*Body composition tests performed by Lovelace Medical Center, Research Division, Albuquerque, New Mexico.

Your reserve fibers participate only when needed. Only the heaviest possible weight will bring the maximum number of muscle fibers into action. Muscle fibers that aren't called on to contract have no reason to grow and get stronger, so they don't.

There's another important aspect to the all-or-none law. A muscle fiber contracts fully or not at all, but the force of the contraction can be weakened by fatigue. If the fatigue is great enough, the fiber can no longer contract. It momentarily loses the ability to contract. It fails.

The number of fibers contracting and the strength of the contraction changes as you perform a set of an exercise. For example, the first repetition of a set may require the contraction of 100 fibers. On the second repetition the 100 fibers lose part of their contractal strength. They can no longer do the job alone. So 10 fresh fibers kick in to exert the additional force needed to lift the weight a second time. On the third repetition the initial 100 fibers, weakened still further, and the 10 additional fibers, now also weakened, can't lift the weight, so more fresh fibers are called into action.

If you stop at that point, you won't give your muscles a reason to get bigger and stronger, because they're still performing well within their normal capacity. But continue to lift the weight as many times as you can, and you'll be in business, the muscle-building business, because now you're forcing all available fibers to contract, and you're completely exhausting at least some of those fibers. You're pushing them to the point of failure. Muscles don't like to be pushed to the limit, so they build a reserve to make it easier next time. They grow bigger and stronger.

Now what do you do to reward your muscles for responding to the challenge? If you want to keep the muscle-building process going, you play a dirty trick on them. Next time you push them even further, to failure again. You force your muscles to build an even greater strength reserve.

Yes, things are tough for the muscles of a bodybuilder. That's what it's all about.

Intensity

"Intensity" is a term used a lot in modern bodybuilding, but it's rarely defined. Like most bodybuilders I knew generally that intensity was a function of hard training, but I had trouble pinning it down more specifically. When my father told me about the all-or-none law, he also told me that the way to get stronger is to continually try to lift heavier weights. He was wiser than I realized at the time. I thought it was interesting that muscle fibers always contract as hard as they can, but I didn't understand what that had to do with attempting weights that I'd never lifted before. Eventually it dawned on me that the all-or-none law explains why training intensity is so important, and why it's essential to keep lifting heavier and heavier weights. When I made the connection between the two concepts, I finally understood the meaning of training intensity.

Intensity is the proportion of available fibers a muscle is using when it contracts. It's the extent to which a muscle is performing to capacity. Maximum training intensity—probably an impossibility—is achieved when *all* available fibers are forced to contract until they fail.

Remember, the brain only calls on the number of muscle fibers it needs. Those muscle fibers contract with all their might, and the remaining muscle fibers do nothing at all. Muscle fibers that aren't used remain small and weak; they fail to develop. If you've ever had an arm or leg in a cast, you know how muscles atrophy (waste away) from lack of use. On the other hand, muscle fibers that are stimulated strongly hypertrophy; they grow bigger and stronger. The fibers themselves get bigger, the stored nutrients increase, and the capillaries supplying blood to the fibers grow in size and number. There's also some evidence that stimulated muscle fibers split and grow in number. This is called hyperplasia.

So the job of the bodybuilder is clear: make as many muscle fibers as possible contract and push the maximum number of those fibers to the point of failure. To make muscles grow and get stronger, the bodybuilder must trigger more and more muscle fibers into action, and force those fibers to work harder than ever before. The bodybuilder must subject his or her muscle fibers to greater and greater training intensity.

Muscle fibers that aren't stimulated remain "off" and underdeveloped. Once I understood this critical corollary to the all-or-none law, I started focusing on training techniques to turn the maximum number of muscle fibers "on."

High-Intensity Techniques

Make the all-or-none law work for you. There are many ways to intensify your training and stimulate more muscle fibers. Your bodybuilding success depends on the number of fibers you trigger into action. Your job is to force more and more fibers to contract harder and harder.

Concentrate—The brain determines the number of muscle fibers to activate for a specific task. That's why it's so important to concentrate on each exercise. Focus on the muscle you're working. Think about the muscle fibers contracting. Don't forget that your brain controls the intensity of your training. It determines how many muscle fibers contract on every repetition of every set. Use your mind to make your muscle fibers come to life and grow. I can't say it better than I did in *Ripped:* "Make the message your brain sends to your muscles a firm command to every muscle fiber to contract and keep contracting until the weight can no longer be lifted."

Lift slowly—If you perform an exercise in a jerky or fast style, you use momentum, not muscle, to lift the weight. Doing an exercise too fast puts stress on the muscle only at the start and the end of the movement. It seriously reduces the quality of the contraction, because you're throwing the weight up and letting it coast through the middle of the movement. On the other hand, performing the exercise smoothly and slowly causes the maximum number of muscle fibers to contract through the full range. Make the muscle fibers contract all the way through the movement, from beginning to end. If you can't feel the muscle contracting throughout the full range, slow down.

Lower Slowly—More weight can be lowered than lifted, and to recruit the maximum number of muscle fibers you must control the weight more while lowering than while lifting. Lowering the weight may actually be more important for strength building than raising it. As a general rule, lowering the weight should take approximately twice as long as lifting it. To activate the maximum number of muscle fibers, be sure you load the muscle through the entire movement, up and down.

Full-Range Contraction—To contract the maximum number of muscle fibers you must stimulate a muscle through its full range of motion, from full extension to full contraction. When you're aware of the need to work a muscle over its full range, it's relatively easy to figure out how to do it.

Take the Standing Barbell Curl, for example. There's little resistance at the beginning and the end of the movement. A lot of muscle fibers are involved only in the middle of the movement. However, you can create resistance at the beginning and end of the curl by using an adjustable preacher curl bench. Move the preacher bench to a 45° angle and you have maximum resistance at the beginning of the movement. At a 90° angle you have maximum resistance at the end of the curl.

Another example is the Dumbbell Side Lateral Raise. When the arm is hanging down there's little resistance. It's only when the arm is extended out to the side that the shoulder muscle, the deltoid, really works. However, if you do the exercise lying on your side, maximum muscle fibers are involved at the start of the movement. Do the movement leaning on an incline bench and you have maximum resistance in the middle range of the movement. It's simply a matter of positioning your body so gravity works for you.

There are also a number of devices that make leverage and gravity work in your favor to create resistance over a muscle's full range of motion. For instance, unlike barbells and dumbbells, a cable threaded through a pulley and attached to a weight stack provides an even resistance as you pull in different directions. The weight stack on a pulley moves straight up and down, no matter what direction you pull the cable, and provides constant resistance throughout the range of movement. I use pulleys to work my chest from different angles. I can contract every part of my pectoral muscle by positioning my body in different ways and using high and low pulleys.

Of course, a number of equipment companies now make machines specifically designed to provide resistance over a full range of movement. Nautilus is the most famous line of full-range machines.

To work my muscles maximally over a full range of motion, I use a combination of free weights, benches, pulleys and machines.

Number of Repetitions—To involve a maximum number of muscle fibers, you must do the proper number of repetitions.

If you perform more than 10 repetitions you'll probably fail because you're out of breath, not because your muscles are exhausted. High repetitions also build up fatigue products which hamper muscle function.

If you perform less than six repetitions you probably won't exhaust a high percentage of muscle fibers. Low repetitions may be good for testing strength, but they're not the best way to build muscular size and strength.

Six to 10 repetitions allows you to stimulate a maximum number of muscle fibers. If I can't do at least six repetitions, I lower the weight. When I can do 10 or more, I raise the weight.

Goals—Before each workout I check my training diary to see what I did the last workout. This gives me a target. I attempt to do a little better than I did the last time. I've found that I work harder if I have a goal to shoot for in each exercise.

After each set, while it's fresh in my mind, I write my goal for the next workout in my training diary. I use a simple system of arrows to indicate whether I should do more repetitions, use more weight, or whatever. When necessary I don't hesitate to repeat a set or even decrease the weight. Goals are no help unless they're realistic. My goal may be simply to lift the same weight for the same number of repetitions, but to do smoother, fuller and better repetitions. That's progress, and progression is always my ultimate goal.

Warm-Up—Don't warm up too much. I only warm up enough to prepare for my heavy set or sets. I never extend myself in warming up, because I want to be strong and fresh for the important set or sets, the heavy ones. I may be able to do 20 repetitions or more with a warm-up weight, but I stop after five or six repetitions. I rarely do more than two warm-up sets. If a similar exercise has prepared me adequately, I skip the warm-up entirely and move directly to my heavy set or sets. In short, I save my energy by only warming up enough to prepare for my heavy sets, no more.

Focus Your Energy—I try to stay fresh throughout my workout so I can exert maximum effort on each exercise. That's why I usually do only one hard set of each exercise. Additional sets use up training energy and reduce the overall intensity of the workout.

I rarely do more than 10 or 12 different exercises in one workout, and I try to make sure that my workouts don't last longer than an hour. I don't rush my workouts at the expense of training intensity. I take enough rest so that I can put maximum effort into the next exercise. I train the largest muscle groups first because they require the greatest energy expenditure. This ensures that I'll be fresh to work each of these muscle groups intensely. For example, I don't train my chest before my legs, or my shoulders and arms before my back.

Overall, the best order to train body parts for maximum intensity is: lower back, legs, upper back, chest, shoulders, arms and abdominals. This order also ensures that you don't weaken the smaller muscle groups that come into play when you're working the larger muscle groups. For instance, it's difficult to train your latissimus dorsi muscle (upper back) if your arms, the link between the lats and the resistance, are tired from doing Curls. Similarly, it's hard to train the chest properly when your triceps or shoulders are tired.

In summary, be careful how you expend your energy. Focus it for maximum intensity.

Cheating, Forced and Negative Repetitions—After I've done as many regular repetitions as I can, I often continue by doing forced repetitions or negative repetitions to involve more muscle fibers and reach a deeper stage of exhaustion. I have a training partner provide just enough assistance so I can "force" a few more repetitions, or the training partner will help me lift the weight so I can continue with the negative part of the exercise, the lowering part, until I can no longer control the weight as I lower it. If no training partner is available, I sometimes loosen my style and do a few cheating repetitions. Like forced or negative reps, cheating allows me to continue beyond normal failure and exhaust more muscle fibers.

Repetition range is important here, too. I'm careful to select a weight that won't allow more than 10-12 total repetitions—regular plus forced, negative or cheating reps. I don't want to become so short of breath that I can't do the cheating, forced or negative repetitions effectively.

Rest-Pause and Negative-Accentuated Repetitions—These two high-intensity techniques can be used without the aid of a training partner.

The rest-pause style allows a series of repetitions with a weight you couldn't lift that many times in regular nonstop style. The advantage is a greater number of near-maximum contractions. This style can be used with most exercises. I especially like it for the Leg Press. I select a weight in the Leg Press that I can raise approximately five times. I lift the weight as many times as I can, rest-pause briefly (about five deep breaths), and then lift the weight again as many times as I can, usually three or four. After another brief pause (a little longer this time), I again do as many repetitions as possible—this time only one or two. When doing the exercise in the regular style, only the last one or two repetitions are "all out." In the rest-pause style, more muscle fibers are involved because a series of near-maximum repetitions are performed back-to-back.

In the negative-accentuated style, the weight is raised with two arms or legs, and lowered with one arm or leg. This style can only be used on machines. I particularly like it for Leg Extensions, Leg Curls, Calf Raises, Pullovers and Curls. Some experts believe that for building strength, lowering the weight is more important than raising it. I'm not sure whether that's true, but judging by the feel in the muscle, the negative-accentuated style produces an extremely good contraction, especially in the fully contracted position. Four to six repetitions with each leg or arm works best for maximum muscle fiber involvement.

One Limb at a Time—Proportionately more weight can be lifted with one arm or leg than with both arms or both legs. If you can curl 100 pounds with two arms, you can probably curl 60 pounds or more using only one arm. The reason is that your brain concentrates the nerve impulse on one limb, rather than dividing it between two limbs. This accounts, in part, for the superior contraction produced by the negative-accentuated style. For the same reason, intensity is increased when you exercise one arm or leg in regular style. Boyer Coe, the 1981 World Grand Prix Champion, has gotten excellent results training one arm or one leg at a time. He's worked up to 10 repetitions with 85 pounds in the One-Arm Side Lateral Raise! This style can be used effectively for almost every body part. The one-limb-at-a-time style is another means of focusing your energy for greater intensity.

Rest Is Important

You can't train too intensely—remember, your objective is to involve and exhaust as many muscle fibers as you can. But you can train too much. It's easy to get carried away by your initial success.

In the beginning almost all bodybuilders have encouraging results. Gains come quick and easy. Weight training in almost any form overloads the muscles and they respond readily. It's normal to think, "If I train more I'll do even better." At this stage bodybuilders are understandably eager. And then they read in one of the muscle magazines that some champion bodybuilders train six days a week, sometimes twice a day. "I knew it!" they say to themselves. And they start working out longer and more often. That's usually a mistake.

Several days ago my wife, my son and I were backsliding a little at the pizza parlor near our house. One of the employees, a young bodybuilder, recognized me. He had the waitress ask me if I was Clarence Bass. A little later, as I was serving myself at the salad bar, he introduced himself and proceeded to tell me that he trains at the YMCA six days a week, two or three hours a day. He said the pictures in the magazines had inspired him. At first he just wanted to "tone up," but now he wanted to "get big." He was puzzled, however, because he wasn't making the progress he expected.

I told him that he was probably training too much. I explained that first he had to stimulate muscle growth by training hard, and then he had to permit growth by resting. He thanked me for the advice. I hope he understood my point. I've had many similar conversations with bodybuilders, young and old. I always emphasize the importance of rest. Muscles can't grow without adequate rest.

I overtrained for years. Former National Coaching Coordinator Carl Miller lives about 60 miles north of me in Santa Fe, N.Mex. Carl and I competed against each other in the National Teenage Olympic Lifting Championship, and we sometimes reminisce about our early training years. Carl has become famous as an Olympic lifting coach. He's written several books and traveled all over the world studying training methods. He maintains that we both would have been better lifters if we had lifted less and rested more. I'm sure he's right.

In our early lifting years, neither of us understood the importance of rest. We both beat our brains out against limit poundages, day after day, and wondered why we weren't improving. Like so many other lifters, then and now, we let our enthusiasm get the best of us.

We're older now, and wiser. Carl proves it by lifting more, in his 40s, than he ever could before. Last year, in 1981, he lifted 281 pounds in the Snatch and 364 in the Clean and Jerk, and he ranked sixth nationally, among light-heavyweight Olympic lifters (181 pounds) of all ages. He lifts more now, in part, because he rests more.

In *Ripped,* I detailed how my progress improved when I changed from long, everyday training sessions to short, hard, infrequent training sessions. Clearly, I do better when I give equal billing in my training to intensity *and* rest.

Training too much and resting too little appears to be a tendency shared by athletes in almost all sports. George Sheehan, the famous runner-doctor, wrote about his own experience in a recent issue of *Runner's World* magazine. He, too, was carried away by his early successes. He ran too fast and too far too often. "I finally realized," he wrote, "that the more I did, the worse I became." Citing stress expert Hans Selye, Sheehan says, "The body can be trained to greater performance by inducing stress. But the amount of stress and the time allowed for recovery are critical to the success of the process."

The ability of the body to recover from exercise is limited. Hard training will get you nowhere in bodybuilding if you don't follow up with enough rest to permit muscle growth to take place. Without adequate rest, your body is forced to use all of its recovery ability just to replace the energy used up in training. For growth to take place, the body must be able to recover the energy expended in training and have enough recovery capacity left over for growth.

I was training with a cold recently, trying to do enough so I wouldn't lose ground, but not make my cold worse. It's an experience I've had many times before—training through a cold. I'll never forget catching cold a few years back, right before a lifting contest. I'd lie flat on my back between training lifts. I wanted to keep working out, but I didn't want to stir up my cold any more than necessary. It was crazy. That's why I remember it so well.

During my bout with this latest cold it occurred to me that the experience of training with a mild illness is a good illustration of limited recovery capacity. Your body is fighting off the illness, so your ability to recover from training is reduced. The difference between training enough to benefit, but not enough to cause a setback, is narrowed. It's a fine line that most athletes have tried to walk. Up to a point you can benefit from exercise, but if you go too far you aggravate your illness. It's a magnified example of recovery capacity.

The same thing applies when you're well. Up to a point the body recovers from exercise and grows stronger. But if you push too much, you exceed your capacity to recover. You won't grow, and if you push even more, you'll actually lose size and strength. Push still more and the result can be exhaustion, illness, and even collapse. Olympic Champion Emil Zatopek expressed it graphically when he said, "[The body] is like a spring—you press and it jumps. You press more and it jumps more. But [training] must be limited so as not to damage the spring."

Bill Bowerman, retired University of Oregon track coach, is considered by many to be the father of the running boom in this country. His book *Jogging,* published in 1967, and his pamphlet with the same title published earlier, started it all. During his years at Oregon, he coached 24 Olympians and guided his school to four NCAA team championships. Bowerman also served as Head Coach for the 1972 U.S. Olympic track team. In a recent interview for *The Runner* magazine, Bowerman put it straight and simple. "Rest is important," he said.

The Hard/Easy Principle

Bill Bowerman's greatest contribution as a coach is probably the hard-day, easy-day training concept. Runners once thought they had to run hard every day, but Bowerman says that every hard day should be followed by an easy day. He believes that overtraining is probably the biggest danger for both joggers and world-class runners. So he teaches that a hard day should be followed by one, two, three or more easy days, until the body is recovered and ready for another hard session.

World-class runner Marty Liquori agrees. He explains in his *Guide for the Elite Runner*: "The idea is simply that one cannot train at 110 percent daily and not expect to end up flat on his or her back after about five days. The body requires both the stress of exercise *and* the serenity of light days in order to grow stronger and faster."

Weightlifters, like runners, used to train hard all the time. But most modern powerlifters and Olympic lifters have learned that hard-day, easy-day training produces better results. Research at Ohio State University has shown that it takes from 48 to 96 hours to recover from high-intensity weight training. Moreover, Dr. David L. Costill, the famous exercise physiologist from Ball State University, has shown that it can take more than five days to restore muscle glycogen used in intense exercise. In actual practice a strong weightlifter may need a week or more to recover and be ready for another maximum-weight workout. This creates a problem, because muscular size and strength begin to decrease after about four days of inactivity. Apparently, the strength of the muscle fibers starts to decline before the glycogen supply is completely restored. Other parts of the body's recovery system, like the adrenal glands, may take more than four days to recuperate as well. The solution? Interposing some lighter workouts which maintain strength without delaying recovery.

Most beginning weightlifters start out training as hard as they can three times a week. This works fine—at first. But as a lifter grows stronger and begins to train harder, greater inroads are made into recovery capacity and it takes longer to recuperate. Eventually it becomes difficult or impossible to recover from more than one or two hard training sessions a week. Doing three or more hard sessions often retards or stops progress.

Most powerlifters find that they can't make gains in a lift if they train heavy in it more than once a week. Dr. Ken Leistner, Feature Editor of *Powerlifting USA* magazine, suggests that powerlifters train each lift a second or third time each week, but with less intensity, to improve technique and prevent atrophy of skeletal muscles.

Four-time world champion Mike Bridges, holder of more world powerlifting records than any other lifter in history, has learned his training tolerance in each of the power lifts. He does a maximum Bench Press on Monday and Friday, but benches light on

Wednesday. He does a 100-percent Squat on Monday, but drops to 50 percent on Wednesday and 75 percent on Friday. It takes a week of complete rest for him to recover from the Deadlift, so he trains that lift only once a week, using maximum weight on Wednesday. Champion powerlifters search until they find the system that works best for them. Their systems vary, but almost without exception, they, like Bridges, use medium and light training days to facilitate recovery and prevent loss of strength.

Champion Olympic lifters structure their training in a similar manner. In his booklet, *Olympic Weightlifting,* former world recordholder Russ Knipp recommends a formula of heavy, medium-heavy, medium and light training. Carl Miller, in his *Olympic Lifting Training Manual,* advocates training loads which vary from 100 percent to 60 percent. Carl tells me that the champion Russian Olympic lifters vary their intensity from light to heavy, with limit lifts spread 10 to 14 days apart.

I believe that bodybuilders, like runners, powerlifters and Olympic lifters, will do best on a heavy-day, easy-day system of training. Study and experimentation over several years have persuaded me to move my training more and more in that direction.

In 1977 I began training for the Past-40 Mr. America on a six-day-a-week split system. I trained my body twice a week, doing up to 20 sets per body part. I trained hard every workout. By 1979, I had reduced my sets to approximately four per body part and adopted a four-day training cycle. I took three days to train my whole body and rested on the fourth day. Compared to 1977, I trained less, but with more intensity. I rested more. I felt better using this system and my results improved—in some cases dramatically (as illustrated by a 44 percent increase in the Leg Press, from 15 repetitions with 450 pounds to 15 repetitions with 650). I continued to train heavy every cycle, however.

In 1980 I began to notice that I wasn't recovering between workouts. Notations of tiredness appeared in my training diary more frequently. I was getting injured more often. A chronic shoulder injury was particularly troublesome. More and more I was finding it necessary to rest an extra day. Finally, as a corrective measure, I started training lighter on some days.

On October 7, 1980, I scribbled a quick note in my training diary: "I think [it would] be better [to] break up [my training cycles] and do regular sets every other time or so—[this will] keep [my] mind fresher and renew enthusiasm." My notation was more cryptic than usual because I was packing for a trip to Belgium as an official with a US team to the European Bodybuilding Championships. A special feature of the contest was a match between the European champions and the American bodybuilders. Jim Manion, President of the National Physique Committee, and I were the officials selected to accompany the US team. Unfortunately, our guys had trouble peaking again so soon after the Mr. America contest. We lost, three classes to one, to the Europeans who were razor sharp for their championship. Nevertheless, the trip was a great experience for me. I hadn't been to Europe before and the Europeans were delightful hosts.

Anyway, that brief note in my training diary signaled the start of my hard-day, easy-day system. In the beginning my "easy" days weren't very easy. My years as an Olympic lifter had exposed me to hard-easy training, but I thought: "Bodybuilders use lighter weights and higher repetitions. They don't need easy-day training." Eventually, I became convinced that was wrong, but my conversion was slow and painful; I resisted all the way.

When I returned from Europe I continued to train my body on a four-day cycle:

Day One	Day Two	Day Three	Day Four
Upper back	Lower back	Traps	Rest
Chest	Legs	Shoulders	
Upper Abs	Obliques	Arms	
		Lower Abs	

The change I made was to vary the intensity of my training from cycle to cycle. On one cycle I trained with maximum intensity, using forced, negative or rest-pause repetitions on most exercises. On the next cycle I omitted the high-intensity techniques and simply trained to positive failure. In other words, on my "easy" days, I trained in regular style, with heavy weights, and did as many repetitions as I could in strict form. Before my trip to Europe, I had been using some combination of forced, negative or rest-pause training in *most* of my workouts.

Finally I had come to realize that my body wouldn't tolerate high-intensity techniques every workout. I found that it helped a lot to back off on my training intensity every other cycle; it made me more enthusiastic on my maximum-intensity days. Mentally, I was more willing to accept forced reps and other high-intensity techniques every other training cycle.

After a while, however, my body told me—through tiredness mostly—that I was still overtraining. Another clue was that I'd find myself stronger in an exercise after I'd skipped that exercise in the previous workout. The extra, unplanned rest had a surprising and telling effect: it made me stronger. As a result of these telltale signals, I began to use less weight and do more repetitions on my regular cycles. I still did almost as many repetitions as I could, however, and I usually couldn't resist doing a few more sets. I called these lighter, high-repetition days "maintenance workouts." Like before, when I'd lightened up by doing "regular" sets every other cycle, these maintenance cycles made my heavy cycles go better. They were a welcome relief, mentally and physically. My muscle response during heavy cycles improved. My body didn't feel "used" all the time. Nevertheless, I still had periods when I was tired or couldn't sleep.

Soon after starting this new system (heavy cycle/maintenance cycle), I hurt my hip doing negative Leg Curls. It was another hint that I wasn't recovering properly. I think the injury was the result of training too much. In fact, I kept writing in my diary that I should lighten up more on my maintenance cycle. But it took another injury to make me actually do it.

I continued alternating cycles until August 1981. On heavy cycles I pushed hard, using high-intensity training techniques. On my maintenance cycles I went as heavy as I could without really straining. My maintenance cycles were still pretty heavy. Using that system I pushed my Leg Press up to 15 repetitions with 700 pounds on August 20, 1981. But on August 23, 1981, I pulled my groin doing one-arm rest-pause repetitions on the pec deck machine. I thought, "That's the end of my Leg Press for a while."

I skipped Leg Presses for 16 days, until September 8, when I tried the exercise again. I made an easy 15 repetitions with 640. My groin felt OK.

Partly as a result of my injury and partly because I simply wanted to try something new, I made another major change in my training system when I started doing Leg Presses again. I started doing "light" cycles in which I would decrease my poundages by 15 to 20 percent with no added repetitions or sets. In other words, I actually started doing easy sets on easy days.

This change brought about a startling result. My leg press

poundage literally shot up. Little more than one month later, on October 16, 1981, I made a lifetime best of 14 repetitions with 750 pounds! In effect, I added 50 pounds to my Leg Press by the simple expedient of resting more. That experience sold me on the hard/easy system of training.

In fact, I might have pushed my leg press record even higher, but a few weeks later the backboard on my leg press machine cracked on my seventh repetition with 770. A pulled groin didn't stop my Leg Press—it actually helped. But the cracked backboard did stop me, at least for the time being.

Here are my leg press poundages as I recorded them in my training diary during the period August 20 to November 4, 1981:

August 20 (Maintenance Cycle)	700 x 15 (Personal best)
August 23	groin injury
August 24 (Hard cycle)	(Injured, skipped Leg Press)
August 31 (Maintenance cycle)	(Injured, skipped Leg Press)
September 8 (Hard cycle) (First workout using the hard-cycle, easy-cycle system)	640 x 15 (was careful to protect groin)
September 12 (Easy cycle)	630 x 10
September 16 (Easy cycle)	640 x 10
September 21 (Hard cycle)	700 x 15
September 25 (Easy cycle)	650 x 10
September 29 (Hard cycle)	750 x 10 (Personal best)
October 3 (Easy cycle)	650 x 10
October 7 (Hard cycle)	750 x 12 (Personal best)
October 12 (Easy cycle)	650 x 10
October 16 (Hard cycle)	750 x 14 (Personal best)
October 20 (Easy cycle)	650 x 10
October 25 (Hard cycle)	760 x 10 (Personal best)
October 30 (Easy cycle)	650 x 10
November 4 (Hard cycle)	770 (Backboard cracked)

So you see, I backed into hard-day, easy-day bodybuilding training, dragging my feet all the way. As I read through my training diary now, I wonder why I was so reluctant to train easy on easy days. Clearly, it works. I'm convinced that the hard-day, easy-day system is the key to my future progress.

At present, I'm experimenting with 70 percent intensity every fourth training cycle. Because, like George Sheehan, I'm realizing that the less I train the better I become.

Listen to Your Body

I haven't always been a Sherlock Holmes in detecting clues of overtraining. It took plain old tiredness, inability to sleep and injuries to make me include easy days in my training. Learn from my experience. Pay close attention to signals from your body. If you let it, your body will tell you whether you're recovering between workouts. Tiredness, insomnia, irritability, depression, hand tremor, loss of appetite and lack of enthusiasm—for training and everything else—are all symptoms of overtraining. If you're not alert to these signs, you can find yourself in deep trouble. Gains stop and, if you keep ignoring your body, exhaustion and illness may follow.

As previously mentioned, an elevated heart rate (five or more beats above normal) when you wake up in the morning is an indication that you haven't recovered from the workouts of the last several days. If that's the case, you should take it easy that day. To detect an elevated heart rate, you must know your normal waking heart rate. Take your pulse for several mornings in a row when you wake up. It's best to lie in bed for a few minutes before taking your pulse, especially if you use an alarm or if something else awakens you suddenly. I always take my pulse by placing my thumb and forefinger on the carotid arteries on the sides of my neck behind my Adam's apple. I usually count for a full minute. A quicker way to do it is to count your pulse for six seconds and add a zero.

When you're trying to judge your recovery it helps to be aware of the "two-day lag." When I was a teenager my doctor father called my attention to the lag between a workout and the time when the full effects are felt. To illustrate, he pointed out that when someone is injured, in a minor auto accident, for instance, the person is stiff and sore the next day, but maximum discomfort usually isn't experienced until the second or third day. Marty Liquori, former American recordholder in the 5000-meter run, discusses this lag in his *Guide for the Elite Runner*: "It usually takes at least one day and more often two for effects (injuries or fatigue) of a hard workout or race to hit you." I almost always feel the most soreness and fatigue two days after a workout. That's when my body really feels used.

If you feel good the day after a hard workout, it doesn't necessarily mean that you're ready for another hard workout. It's best to wait another day. Take the two-day lag into account when planning and evaluating your workouts. Build rest into your schedule. That's what Coach Bowerman's easy-day, hard-day principle is all about.

Experiment and learn your recovery capacity and your response to work loads. Your body will tell you when it's time to let up. Listen to it.

Coaxing Long-Term Gains

The 18th century British statesman Edmund Burke said, "The use of force alone is but temporary." He was talking about relations with colonial America, but that statement could apply to bodybuilding as well.

Gains in muscular size and strength can only be forced temporarily. Long-term gains must be coaxed. "To coax" means to induce in an agreeable manner, by gentle persuasion. Few bodybuilders are willing or able to strain to the limit continually. I doubt that anyone really wants to do Curls, or any other exercise, until they're blue in the face, not on a regular basis anyway. The mind rebels. It won't face such effort day after day. What's more, I don't think it's necessary or, in the long run, desirable. I look on bodybuilding as a lifetime pursuit, a pursuit to be enjoyed, not suffered.

Don't misunderstand, I try hard in the gym; but I don't continually butt my head against the wall. True, I constantly try to lift more. But rather than concentrate on getting out every last repetition in every workout, I focus on progression. The essence of successful bodybuilding is progression, and long-term progression comes through patience and moderation, not force.

Let me explain. From the physiological standpoint, absolute, gut-busting, maximum effort is the best way to induce muscular gains, but like the song goes, "You got to know when to hold 'em, know when to fold 'em, know when to walk away and know when to run." Bodybuilding progress, like progress in any other activity, is irregular; it's full of peaks, valleys and plateaus. Don't expect to make continuous progress. A bodybuilder should push for a while, back off, and then push again. Sticking points are inevitable.

When you've reached a sticking point, the traditional advice is to take a brief layoff, change the exercise, increase the weight or decrease the weight. Those are good suggestions, but there are other strategies which help to ensure continued progress. I've already discussed some of these strategies: hard-easy training, workout-to-workout training goals and listening to your body for signs of overtraining. But it's even more important that you take a long-term approach to training. Plan your routine on a yearly basis. Plan to improve every year, but don't expect to improve every month.

Runners and athletes in other sports don't try to stay in top shape all the time. Bodybuilders shouldn't either. I make a push each year for six to nine months. Generally, I train moderately hard for about six months, and then I work very hard for an additional three months to reach peak form. After I peak, I take it easy. I spend about three months each year letting my body recuperate, just recharging, physically and mentally, to push again the next year.

Most athletes follow a similar pattern. Peak form can't be maintained. In fact, attempting to stay in peak form will limit your progress. Peak form is, by definition, temporary. What goes up must come down. An athlete maintains a peak for a short time, and then comes down. A condition that can be maintained isn't peak condition. The body can be pushed to a peak, but then it must rest.

Frank Zane says he begins his serious training every year as a beginner. He peaks for the Mr. Olympia contest, and then takes it easy. He builds up every year, and every year he gets better. Even Mike Mentzer, bodybuilding's number one advocate of high-intensity training, reserves his most intense workouts for contest preparation. He knows he can't train hard all year.

In 1982 the great miler Sebastian Coe was aiming for the European Championships and the Commonwealth Games scheduled for September and October. "I don't want to be fit too early," he said in an interview. "I don't want to reach anything like a peak before the beginning of August."

Take a tip from champion athletes like Frank Zane, Mike Mentzer and Sebastian Coe: give your body a break every year. Expect ups and downs in your training. Indeed, plan for them.

You should also take a similar long-range view from workout to workout. In 1981 I made it a point to coax my body, not force it. To lift the most at the end of the season, I decided to stop a little short of my limit each workout. This was a change of strategy. In 1980 I pushed as hard as possible every workout. I squeezed out every last repetition that I could. I left every session satisfied that I'd done my best. But I also carried away a nagging doubt: can I do more next time? Constant forcing in this way brought on premature sticking points. I failed to reach goals I knew were within my capacity.

In 1981 I held back slightly each workout. I pushed hard, but not to the ragged edge. Nevertheless, I made it a point to lift a little more weight or do another repetition or two each workout. I increased the weight continuously, but not enough to stall my progress. My poundage increases were moderate and gradual. I passed up short-term gains in favor of uninterrupted progress. Instead of large poundage increases daily, my goal was long-term progress. I maintained a reserve of strength to build on. Stopping just short of my limit and increasing the weight in small increments gave me confidence for my next workout. The mental hazard created by butting up against my absolute limit each time was avoided. I went into each workout with a positive attitude. I knew I could do more, and I did, workout after workout.

In 1980, during a 4½-month peaking period, I got stuck in the Leg Press seven times. In 32 workouts I was able to increase the weight only seven times. One sticking point lasted 1½ months.

By contrast, in 1981, I didn't hit a single sticking point. during my 11-week peaking period, from June 7 to August 24, I increased my leg press poundage every workout—19 straight increases without a failure! Coaxing my gains in 1981 paid off in continuous progress and more strength.

To gain muscular size and strength, you must lift progressively heavier weights. You'll progress further, however, workout to workout, and year to year, through moderation and patience. Don't force it. Coax it.

Muscle-Building Nutrition

The three basic requirements for building muscle are: 1) High-intensity exercise, 2) Adequate rest and 3) Proper nutrition. Proper nutrition is a key component of the muscle-building process, but it's a component that's widely misunderstood.

Contrary to popular belief, high-intensity exercise doesn't tear down muscle tissue, and no extra protein is needed to rebuild muscle following exercise. You may have read that protein is muscle fuel. That's not true. Dr. Nathan J. Smith, in his excellent book

78

Food for Sport, says, "It is important for athletes to recognize that their athletic activity, although it may require a high energy expenditure, will not significantly increase their need for protein."

Actually, protein is the least efficient source of energy. The main fuel for muscles is carbohydrate, which is available in the blood as glucose and is stored in the muscles and liver in the form of glycogen. The quick energy needed for high-intensity weight training comes primarily from the breakdown of glycogen into the blood sugar, glucose. The body stores of glycogen are limited and must be constantly replenished, especially following intense exercise. If intense exercise is continued for long periods, the stored glycogen in the muscles can be completely depleted.

Recovery following exercise depends primarily on the restoration of glycogen stores in the muscles. And the speed of the recovery depends largely on what you eat following exercise. A diet high in carbohydrate speeds the restoration process. On the other hand, a diet high in protein and fat, and low in carbohydrate, slows the rate of recovery. In fact, a high fat and protein diet may be no better than fasting for recovery purposes. Studies have shown that a high carbohydrate diet fully restored the glycogen in the muscles after 48 hours, while a high protein and fat diet left glycogen levels below par even after five full days. Clearly, a diet high in carbohydrate does the best job of getting you ready for your next workout.

It may surprise you to learn that muscle tissue is mostly water, about 70 percent, and only about 20 percent protein. Drinking water doesn't cause muscles to become larger and consuming extra protein doesn't either. Only a little more than the usual amount of protein is required for muscle-building purposes. Muscle building is a slow process. The amount of muscle that can be added each day is so small that very little extra protein is needed. The protein supplied by a well-balanced diet is almost always sufficient.

At one time I shared the view that the Recommended Daily Allowance (RDA) for protein prepared by the National Research Council was probably inadequate for a bodybuilder trying to add muscle. I changed my mind after I studied the basis for the Research Council's recommendation on protein.

Not only is the Council composed of a large number of respected nutrition scientists, its recommendations take into account the great variations of individual needs and actually are set higher than the needs of most people. The RDA for protein is based on nitrogen balance studies. "Positive nitrogen balance" occurs if we take in more protein than we lose. It means that growth is occurring. "Negative nitrogen balance" means that we're losing more protein than we're taking in and, therefore, that we're not getting enough protein; we're discarding more protein tissue than we're replacing.

Nitrogen balance studies show that a man weighing 154 pounds loses 23 grams of protein daily. This means that he needs 23 grams of protein each day to stay even, i.e., .32 grams of protein for each kilogram of body weight (about .15 grams for each pound). However, the National Research Council doesn't set its RDA for protein at 23 grams daily for a 154-pound man. It allows for protein digestion problems, dietary stresses and other possible problems. The Council sets its RDA for protein at a point high enough to provide for the rare person whose needs are unusually high. The most recent official figures from the National Research Council are *70 grams* of protein for a 154-pound man (one gram for each 2.2 pounds of bodyweight). The average person probably needs only .32 grams of protein for each kilogram of bodyweight, so the RDA of one gram per kilogram provides a wide safety margin for muscle building. The hard training bodybuilder needs extra carbohydrates for energy, but it's extremely unlikely that he or she needs more than one gram of protein for each 2.2 pounds of bodyweight.

As you know from reading Part One of this book, my daily intake of high-quality protein foods is about one quart of milk or yogurt, an occasional egg and a little of my own brand of protein supplement. My other protein comes from foods which individually do not contain all of the essential amino acids, but when eaten in combination do provide complete protein: beans, nuts, seeds, grains and vegetables. Normally I consume approximately 40 grams of high-quality protein—milk and yogurt mainly. Then lower quality protein foods—peanut butter, beans, rice, oats, bread and potatoes—bring my protein intake up to or above the one gram per 2.2 pounds of bodyweight recommended by the National Research Council.

It's important to understand that there's no need to eat a great deal of extra food of any kind—protein, fat or carbohydrate—when you're trying to gain muscle. In fact, calories much beyond those necessary to maintain your body weight will almost always be added in the form of fat. On the rare occasions when I make a conscious effort to gain weight, I'm careful not to add more than 100-200 extra calories, the number supplied by one or two eggs a day. This is a significant point. Don't make the mistake of stuffing down extra food when you're trying to gain muscle. Invariably the result will be added fat, not muscle.

Calorie intake is probably more critical when you're trying to lose weight than when you're trying to gain. It's a mistake to cut calories so severely that you don't supply the energy needed to train hard and, therefore, protect your existing muscle tissue. Remember, you'll lose muscle fibers that you don't use. If you lose more than two pounds of body weight a week, you're almost sure to lose muscle tissue. The calorie deficit required to lose more than two pounds a week reduces your energy supply too much; it makes you too tired to train properly. The bottom line is: if you deviate too far from your maintenance calorie requirements, up or down, you'll gain fat or lose muscle.

A balanced diet of natural foods is best whether you're trying to gain or lose. Eat *slightly* less when you're trying to lose and *slightly* more when you're trying to gain.

When you eat is also important. In his book *Medical Advice for Runners,* Dr. George Sheehan makes a point worth noting. Sheehan's primary demand of diet is that it not interfere with his running. He always runs on an empty stomach and colon. That's good advice for bodybuilders as well. You can't train properly with a stomach or intestinal tract full of food; it makes breathing difficult and diverts blood from the muscles to the digestive tract.

I solve this problem by training in the morning before breakfast. About 30 minutes before my workout I have a piece of fruit (usually a banana). This light snack keeps me from feeling hungry without interfering with my workout. It elevates my blood sugar and prepares me to start training. My main source of workout energy comes from food eaten over the last several days, however. A pre-workout meal can't be digested and converted to glycogen fast enough to supply much energy. Glycogen is restored to the liver after one or two meals, but research has shown that it takes 48 hours or more to restore the glycogen to depleted muscles.

If I find it necessary to train later in the day, I try to eat two or three hours beforehand. It takes at least that long for a meal to empty out of the stomach and upper small intestine. I've trained within an hour after eating, but I prefer to wait longer. I stick with easy-to-digest carbohydrate foods—fruit, vegetables and whole grains—and avoid foods high in fats and proteins. A meal high in protein and fat, especially meat, can take 10-12 hours to empty into the intestine. Examples of easy-to-digest pre-workout meals are: baked potato and yogurt, or cereal with skimmed milk and a banana.

Finally, it's best to spread your meals throughout the day. My pattern of three main meals plus several snacks provides me with a steady source of energy for training and other activities. It keeps my blood sugar level on an even keel and keeps me from getting hungry. I'm less inclined to overeat when I spread my meals out over the course of a day.

Spreading your calories out over the day is especially important when you're trying to add muscle without fat. Some bodybuilders prepare for competition by eating one big meal and fasting the rest of the day. Recently I read about a California competitor who lost 15 pounds in a week by eating only one piece of fruit and a six-ounce can of low sodium tuna before his daily workout. That was it. The only other thing he consumed was distilled water. He became incredibly cut, and he won the contest. I can't argue with his results, but I do wonder what happened to his bodyfat level after the contest when he went back to regular eating.

In his book *Fit or Fat?*, Covert Bailey reports an experiment with rats which shows that eating only one big meal a day can lead to a big fat gain when normal eating is resumed. Two groups of rats were fed the same low-calorie diet, but one group was given only 30 minutes to eat. The other group was allowed to nibble throughout the day. When the rats were allowed to return to a normal amount of food, both groups gained weight. However, the group that had been eating one big meal a day gained more weight than the nibblers.

Bailey explains that the fat-depositing enzymes in the group that ate one big meal increased nearly tenfold during the low-calorie diet. The nibblers had no increase in fat-depositing enzymes. Bailey says that it was as if the bodies of the "One Big Mealers" were saying, "The minute more food comes along, I'm ready to lay down extra fat just in case this stress happens to me again!" The stress, of course, was being deprived of food each day for over 23 hours. So it seems that if you want to gain muscle and not fat, it's important you give your body a small but steady supply of food.

Now let's sum up muscle-building nutrition. A well-balanced diet which supplies your energy needs is all that's required to build muscle. Spread your meals out over the course of the day, but don't eat too close to workouts. Remember, excess calories from any source build fat, not muscle. Don't force down extra protein. Don't restrict carbohydrates. And don't overeat.

Active Rest

My daily walks do more than burn calories; they help me recuperate from workouts as well. Intense weight training causes a rapid buildup of waste products, especially lactic acid, in the muscle. My walks help me get rid of the lactic acid in my muscles.

If sufficient oxygen is present during exercise, glycogen in the muscles is broken down completely and the by-products, water and carbon dioxide, are carried off. It's a clean process. Nothing is left over to impair muscle function.

During light or moderate exercise, like walking or jogging, the heart and lungs can deliver enough oxygen to burn glycogen completely. Energy is produced aerobically (with oxygen). But during intense exercise, like weight training, the body can't keep up with the oxygen demand and muscle cells are forced to work anaerobically—i.e., without the benefit of oxygen. When glycogen is broken down anaerobically, the process isn't complete and lactic acid accumulates. The buildup of waste products causes fatigue and, eventually, further exercise becomes impossible.

Lactic acid remains in the muscles until more oxygen is pumped in, allowing it to be burned aerobically. Runners are urged to "cool down" after a race by walking or jogging a few miles to work the waste products out of their muscles and speed recovery. I do the same thing after my weight workouts. I take a recovery walk.

I follow almost every workout with a two- or three-mile walk (40 minutes to an hour). The gentle aerobic stimulation of walking helps my muscles get rid of waste products faster. It relieves stiffness and soreness, and speeds recovery. In the past I did nothing after workouts and relied on normal activity to burn off the lactic acid in my muscles. I find I recover faster when I walk after workouts.

Recovery walks work best immediately after a workout. If I train in the morning and wait until evening to walk, the waste products seem to settle in my muscles, and it's harder to get rid of the soreness and stiffness. Even if I wait only an hour, the walk doesn't help as much.

If I'm pressed for time, if the weather makes walking uncomfortable, or if I simply don't feel like walking, I ride my stationary bicycle for up to 30 minutes after my workout. Walking is more relaxing and seems to work better, but stationary biking does the job, too.

Try active rest—walking, jogging or biking—after training. You'll find it a pleasant way to bridge the gap between your workout and the rest of the day. The day goes better and so does the next training session.

Combining Weight Training and Aerobics

To burn fat and keep fit, bodybuilders often include an aerobic activity like running or biking in their program. Weight training and aerobics are an ideal combination. Weight training is the best way to build strength and muscle, and aerobic exercise is the best way to develop cardiovascular fitness. The combination can cause problems, however. Overtraining, according to track coach Bill Bowerman and Dr. David L. Costill, world-renowned researcher in the physiology of distance running, is probably the greatest single error made by runners. Bike riders have the same problem. Bodybuilders frequently train too much as well. The trick is to get the benefit of both disciplines without overdoing it. Too much weight training hurts the performance of a runner or a cyclist. Likewise, aerobic exercise can interfere with a bodybuilder's progress.

I don't run because I don't like the pounding on my back and knees, but I do ride a bike. Through trial and error, I've developed some guidelines that allow me to engage in aerobic exercise without hindering my bodybuilding.

First, bodybuilding is my primary activity. I keep that in mind when I plan my bike rides. I always do my weight training before I bike. My first priority is that I be fresh for my bodybuilding workouts. Biking comes second.

It's easy for bike riding to get in the way of leg training in the gym. If the glycogen in the leg muscles is depleted from bike riding, you can't do justice to Squats and other leg exercises. To avoid this problem I schedule my hard bike rides carefully. I've found that the best time for a hard bike ride is on leg training day. I train my legs, and then I take my hard bike ride. This allows me to recover from biking before I train my legs again. It works better than training legs one day, and riding the bike hard the next. It also works better than riding the bike on my rest day. My rest day is for recuperation from weight training, not the time to wear myself out with other activities. Again, it's a matter of priorities. I don't want to be dragging during my leg training sessions. I'd rather start my bike ride a little tired.

Generally, hard bike riding isn't compatible with hard weight training. I've tried charging up hills on a bike and doing 20-mile rides for time. It doesn't work—if weight training is your number one priority. I still ride my bike hard, but only occasionally (about once every eight to 12 days). Experience has taught me how much I can ride my bike without interfering with my bodybuilding. Doing a moderate 30-minute bike ride, stationary or moving, five or six days a week keeps me fit without hampering my weight training. Unless you plan to race, it's not necessary to do more.

Experiment and find out what works for you. Monitor how you feel. Watch for the symptoms of overtraining: restless sleep, loss of appetite, reduced performance and elevated resting heart rate.

Remember, rest is essential for progress both in weight training and aerobic exercise. They're a fine combination, but too much of a good thing causes trouble.

The Best Time of Day to Train

Bodybuilding has its "early birds" who train first thing in the morning and its "night owls" who train as late as midnight—or even later. The famous Jack LaLanne jumps out of bed before dawn to train. Four-time Mr. Universe Bill Pearl does the same thing. Training early worked well for Bill during the years that he operated his very successful gym in California. It continues to work well for him in Oregon where he now conducts his equally successful mail order business.

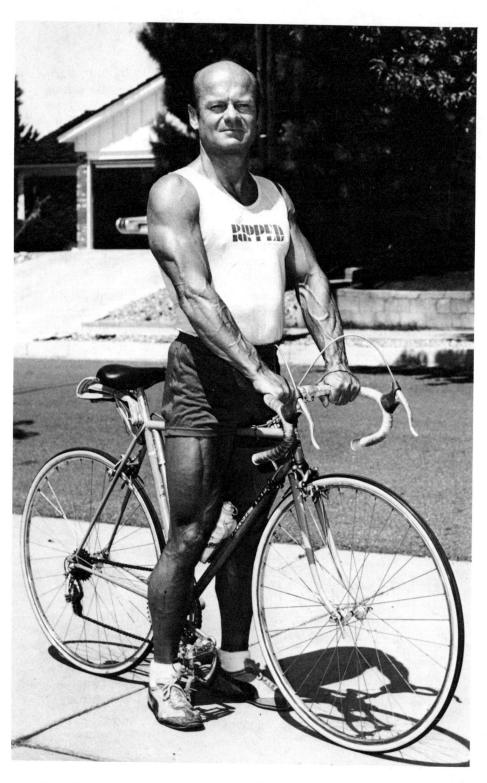

I combine biking with my weight training, but I'm careful not to overdo it. *Photo by Bill Reynolds.*

Pete Grymkowski, Mr. World and the owner of Gold's Gym, trains in the middle of the night. "I am at my physical best between midnight and 6 a.m.," he says. Like Pearl, Pete is too busy to train during the day. The middle of the night is the only time when he can be sure of being able to train without constant interruptions.

Boyer Coe, who has won more top titles than any other bodybuilder, has also trained during the middle of the night. Before moving to California from Louisiana, Boyer operated a health food store and gym, which forced him to train after midnight.

Two-time Mr. Olympia Franco Columbu, a chiropractor, falls between the two extremes. He structures his office hours and his other responsibilities so he can train in the late morning before lunch.

Most bodybuilders probably train in the late afternoon or early evening. It's simply a matter of convenience. That's when they get off work. Obviously, successful bodybuilders train at every hour of the day and night. Still, is there an ideal time to train?

Charted body rhythms suggest certain times of the day are better for training than others. Body temperature systematically rises and falls during the day. The rate of temperature change is small, about a degree and a half. Nevertheless, the fluctuation represents a significant change in the body's metabolic rate.

Science writer Jonathan B. Tucker reports that "a person's hours of peak performance on tasks requiring muscular coordination are likely to coincide with the time of highest body temperature, in the late afternoon or evening. Worst performance occurs at the time of lowest body temperature, in the early morning, when the body is apt to be asleep and the musculature relaxed."

Tucker says that skeletal muscle tone also changes during the day: it's poorest early in the morning when the basal metabolic rate is low. For this reason, many athletes have found that injuries are more common early in the morning, when muscles, joints and tendons are stiff. Dr. Donald LaSalle, director of the Talcott Mountain Science Center in Avon, Conn., studied changes in hand grip strength during the day. Again, the worst performance was early in the morning. Best performances were in the latter half of the day, between 12:30 and 7 p.m.

It seems that the body is most receptive to training in the afternoon or early evening. When marathon runner Bill Rodgers was a teacher he trained at 6 a.m. When he began to make his living through running and could structure his day around it, he switched to the early afternoon. "I've always felt that those 6 a.m. training runs I used to do when I was a teacher weren't the best way to make the Olympic team," he said in a recent issue of *The Runner* magazine.

If you're like Bill Rodgers and can structure your day around your training, then you should train in the afternoon or early evening. Most of us, however, have to make do by squeezing our training into our other activities, whether or not it suits our body rhythms. We're more like Bill Rodgers, the teacher, than Bill Rodgers, the runner.

Boyer Coe says that you can make good gains no matter what time you train. If you're motivated, you can make your body perform in the morning, the afternoon, the evening or even in the middle of the night. Boyer should know. He's trained at all hours of the day and night. If you have to, you can overcome your biological rhythms and get the job done.

I haven't tried training in the middle of the night—I'll leave that to Pete and Boyer—but I have trained at just about every other time. On weekends I've often trained in the early afternoon. That's probably the ideal time of day to train. However, during the week my office hours usually have prevented me from training in the early afternoon. So for most of my bodybuilding career I usually trained in the evening after dinner. I thought it probably would have been better to train before dinner, but my appetite usually got the best of me. This created problems, because after dinner I felt like sitting down and relaxing. It was always hard to get back up again and train. Another problem was that I couldn't control my activities during the day. I often came home from the office feeling tired and strung out. This made it even harder to get up after dinner and train.

The evening just isn't a good time for me to train. My daily activities usually sap my enthusiasm for training, at least to some extent. My wife, Carol, also finds it difficult to train in the evening, but for different reasons. She's away from home all day and wants to take care of household activities in the evening and, more importantly, to spend time with our son, Matt. It's hard for her to concentrate on training when she feels she's neglecting her other responsibilities. I suspect that many other men and women encounter similar problems with evening training.

In May 1981, I was in northern California for the Jr. USA

physique contest. I took the opportunity to go farther north and visit Bill and Judy Pearl at their new headquarters in Oregon. This gave me the opportunity to sample early morning training with Bill. Pearl picked me up at the airport at about 9 o'clock in the evening. We went directly to his home, where Judy was waiting up to greet me. She was "waiting up" because she and Bill go to bed early so they can get up early to train. I was aware that Bill trained early in the morning, but I was shocked when he handed me an alarm clock set for 4 a.m.! I knew I could make myself get up at 4 a.m.— especially to train with Bill Pearl—but I wondered if I could train effectively at that hour.

Well, I was sleeping soundly in the Pearl guest house when the alarm went off. About 30 minutes later I followed Bill out the back door and up the steps to the building which houses his home gym. He had to tell me how many paces it was between steps so I wouldn't stumble in the darkness.

To my surprise I found that training before dawn was OK. With the help of two big cups of coffee, my body was awake and ready to follow Bill through his workout. I felt surprisingly good throughout the training session, which lasted about two hours. I yawned a little the rest of the day, but otherwise I felt all right. The next morning I got up at 4 a.m. and trained with Bill a second time. Again, I felt surprisingly good throughout the workout.

When I got back home I began to consider switching my training time from evening to early morning. I thought back to my law school years, when I broke up my study time by going to bed early, and then got up early to hit the books for several more hours before I went to class. This worked extremely well. Once I was up, there was nothing else to do but study. Through three years of law school I went to bed early and got up at about 4 a.m. to study. I suppose it was an odd schedule, but it worked.

I asked Carol if she wanted to try early morning training to see how it would go. She thought about it for a while and finally said, "OK, let's try it." We've now been getting up early to train for over a year. In 30 years of training, it's the best timetable I've ever tried. I intend to continue early morning training indefinitely (or at least until I figure out how to become more like Bill Rodgers, the runner, than Bill Rodgers, the teacher).

It does take a while to adjust to early morning training and sometimes going to bed early is inconvenient. It doesn't do much for one's social life. Another problem is the telephone. People don't know (or don't believe) we go to bed between eight and nine. Sometimes we're forced to take the phone off the hook.

On the other hand, one of the best things about early morning training is that there are no distractions and no interruptions. My training sessions are consistently good. I'm not tired from working all day, so I'm fresh for every workout. Sometimes I have to stretch and do a few deep knee bends to wake up, but after I get going I'm fine. I have no trouble exerting maximum effort early in the morning. My muscle response is good and injuries haven't been a problem. Best of all, I don't have to train after dinner when I feel more like sitting down or going to sleep. On balance, early in the morning is the best time for me to train.

It boils down to this: physiologically, the best time to train is in the afternoon or early evening. But, if necessary, you can overcome your body rhythms and make good gains at any time that fits your lifestyle. LaLanne, Pearl, Grymkowski, Columbu, Coe and others have worked out their special training time puzzle. You can, too.

The Age Factor

The newspaper headline made me mad. "Age Ends Ali Career," it read. Thirty-nine-year-old Muhammad Ali had just lost a unanimous decision to Trevor Berbick. In *Sports Illustrated* about a week later, Ali was quoted as saying, "I think I'm too old. I was slow. I was weak. Nothing but Father Time." Yes, it made me mad. Why was age the lead item in the stories about Ali's poor showing? Why didn't the media headline Ali's weight and lack of training instead? Less than two months earlier Ali had arrived at his training camp weighing 249 pounds. Apparently, he walked through his roadwork. He weighed in for the fight at a paunchy 236¼. The fat hung on his sides in folds. Was age really the main factor in his defeat? I doubt it.

A week or so earlier former champion Joe Frazier stumbled through a comeback bid against someone named Jumbo Cummings and lost a split decision. You guessed it. The headline began "37-year-old Joe Frazier..." The follow-up story in *Sports Illustrated* called Frazier an old man who "hadn't eluded the inexorable march of time." Buried in the deep recesses of the story was the fact that

Frazier weighed in at 229, 23½ pounds more than when he beat Ali in 1971. Frazier looked like an old man all right, a *fat* old man. He looked like he swallowed a medicine ball. Did age beat Joe Frazier? Again, I doubt it.

The press would have us believe that after age 30 it's downhill all the way. *Esquire* magazine recently cataloged the toll the years take. We're told that after 30, we die a little every day, that we lose about one percent of our functional capacity every year. At age 30, the lines start to form on our foreheads and our hearing starts to go. At 40, we're getting shorter in height, our waist begins to balloon and our stamina is definitely on the decline. At 50... well, you get the idea. *Esquire* says there's no good evidence that exercise slows the aging process. The best strategy, they suggest, is "to relax, hope you have the right genes, and accept peacefully the indignities as they occur." Hell, at almost 45, I'd better hang up my posing trunks and trade in my weights on a rocking chair.

Happily, some experts tell a different story. Exercise physiologist David L. Costill, Ph.D., Director of the Human Performance Laboratory at Ball State University, says the easy chair is not the answer. "If a middle-aged adult wants to become physically active, his muscles are just as adaptable as a teenagers," Costill says. "People in their 50s can go into training and get into better shape than most 20-year-olds."

Bodybuilding has plenty of examples to back up Dr. Costill's position on exercise and aging. Ed Corney, the 1972 Mr. Universe, is still holding his own with the top professional bodybuilders at age 50. The 1951 Mr. America, Roy Hilligenn, made a comeback a few years ago and made a great impression on the judges at the Mr. International contest. He was 54. Bill Pearl posed at the 1978 Mr. America contest to celebrate the 25th anniversary of his 1953 Mr. America win. Had he entered he might have won. He looked great! In 1981 Pearl gave an exhibition in Australia at the Professional Mr. Universe contest. On the eve of his 52nd birthday he fit right in with pros 20 years or more his junior.

Actually, many bodybuilders don't reach top form until they're over 40. Pearl was probably at his all-time best when he won the Professional Mr. Universe contest in 1971. He challenged every bodybuilder in the world to compete against him at that time, and he won. He was 41. Chris Dickerson was 40 years old when he won the overall Grand Prix title in 1980. At 41, Dickerson placed second in the Mr. Olympia contest. The 1982 Pro World Champion, Albert Beckles, is 46. Beckles is unquestionably better than ever. "I do not accept the fact of age," he says. "I train now just as I have always trained—to get better."

Don't misunderstand; there's no getting around the fact that age is a factor. But it's not as much a factor as we're generally led to believe. We don't have to decline by 10 percent for each decade after age 30.

Addressing the subject of aging in his medical advice column in *Runner's World* magazine, Dr. George Sheehan pointed out recently that the generally accepted nine to 10 percent decline per decade is based on misleading data. It's based on people who do nothing to stay young in function, and it doesn't distinguish between pure aging and the decline that comes from disuse.

Dr. Sheehan is presently part of a study designed to measure the rate of decline in athletes who continue to train for peak performance. The rate of deterioration for this group is about five percent per decade, one-half the usually quoted rate. In support of this slower rate of decline, Dr. Sheehan points out that the world marathon record for 40-year-olds is within five minutes of the world record. Sheehan himself, at over 60, can still run the mile in five minutes and 10 seconds, only 20 percent slower than his best college time of 4:20.

Dr. Michael Pollock, an exercise physiologist and Director of the Center for Evaluation of Human Performance at Mount Sinai Medical Center in Milwaukee, is conducting the study in which Dr. Sheehan is a subject. He's finding that we don't have to passively endure the aging process. We can do something about it.

Dr. Pollock has been studying 24 world-class masters runners since 1971. They currently range in age from 50-82. Eleven of them have continued to compete at a very high level, but some of the others haven't maintained their training intensity. This variation has given Dr. Pollack a unique opportunity to measure the difference in the rate of aging based on how much training a person is doing.

There's a significant difference. Dr. Pollock's measurements of aging—body weight, lean body mass, percentage of body fat, lung capacity, blood pressure, resting and maximum heart rate, and maximum oxygen uptake—show a marked decline when training intensity drops off. Those who continued to train hard, Dr. Pollock

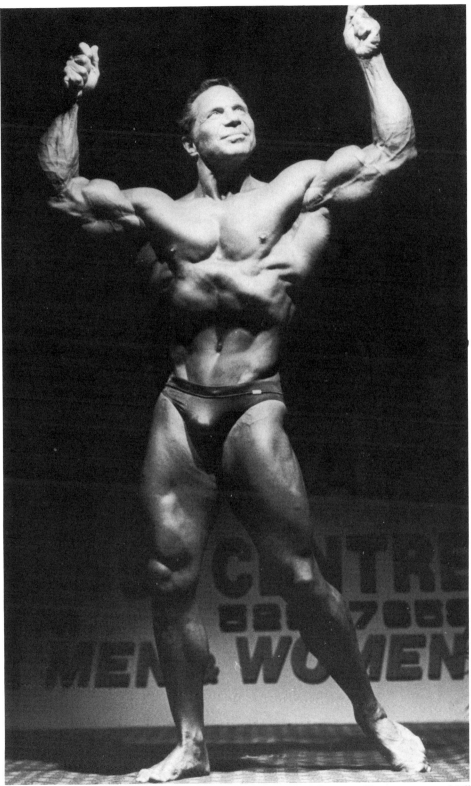

51-year-old Bill Pearl at the 1981 Professional Mr. Universe Contest. *Photo courtesy of Bill Pearl.*

says, showed much less deterioration from aging. In fact, some of them showed no decline at all.

For example, Hal Higdon, author of the excellent book *Fitness After Forty* (World Publications, 1977) and a world masters champion, didn't seem to age. In 1971 he ran a 2:40 marathon at age 41; in 1981 he ran a 2:29 marathon at age 50. Dr. Pollock tested Higdon three time, in 1971, 1976 and 1981. Here are the results as published in *Running* magazine:

	1971	1976	1981
Maximum oxygen uptake	62.7	69.4	63.2
Maximum heart rate	160	160	160
Resting heart rate	34	32	33
Percentage of body fat	10.9	9.5	10.3

Obviously, Higdon has been training regularly, hard and intelligently.

One of Dr. Pollock's findings is of special interest to bodybuilders. His subjects lost muscle mass, even when they kept running. "It doesn't appear that running itself is enough to maintain lean body mass," Pollock says. "It only maintains leg muscles. It doesn't work on total muscle mass." An overall exercise, like weight training, is necessary to maintain muscle mass.

Personally, I intend to do my best to hold out against aging. In fact, I'm going to try to get better. I know the aging process will eventually get me, but I'm going to put up a fight. Dr. Pollock says, "If a person stays injury-free and can stay motivated, the changes of aging can be held off for a long time." I believe him, and I plan to back up that belief with action.

After all, I've got more to gain now, at almost 45, than when I was younger. Swimmer Gail Roper, who is faster at 52 than she was at 18 and holds 43 national masters records, told it like it is in *Sports Illustrated:* "When your body starts to deteriorate, that's when you have to exercise and take care of it to improve the quality of your life."

At this point, I'd be remiss if I failed to include a note of caution. If you're out of shape and want to start training, you should take the advice of the American Medical Association: *"Start slowly* and increase the vigor and duration of the activity as your fitness improves." If you have health problems, you should see your doctor before starting an exercise program. If you're over 40 and you haven't been exercising, it would be a good idea to check with your doctor in any event.

A final comment, probably the most important one of all: you can benefit from exercise at any age. Go for it.

Women Bodybuilders

Women bodybuilders are serious about what they're doing. If I didn't know that already, I knew it when Bill Pearl led me up the steps to his home gym, before dawn, and I learned that his training partner is a woman. Ann Summers walked in right behind us. She went through the workout with us, set for set and rep for rep. She helped Bill with his forced reps and he helped her. The next morning Ann did 25 sets of Chin-Ups with Bill and me. I was impressed. I'd never seen a woman train that hard before. I guess I was a little too enthusiastic, because my wife tells me now that when I got home she got damned tired of hearing about Bill Pearl's training partner. Yes, no doubt about it, in the 1980s women are serious about bodybuilding.

Such zeal wasn't always so common. In the early '50s, when I started training, Abbye "Pudgy" Stockton was featured in *Strength & Health* magazine from time to time. She was strong and had a good figure. Obviously, Pudgy was serious about her training. At the time, she was an oddity, one of a kind. In 1956 Vera Christensen began her "To the Ladies" column in *Strength & Health* magazine. It's still a regular feature. Vera was, and is, serious about bodybuilding for women, but she has never stressed the competitive aspect of the sport.

But in the late 1970s Lisa Lyon, impressed by Arnold Schwarzenegger, joined Gold's Gym and took up bodybuilding with a vengeance. A short time later she emerged from Gold's to become the first World Woman's Bodybuilding Champion. Lisa created a new standard of muscle and beauty for women. She attracted the attention of women everywhere. She captured their imagination. She opened the floodgates. Since then, women's bodybuilding has exploded on the scene.

Virtually every woman's magazine has jumped on the bandwagon. They've started carrying articles on bodybuilding for women. Women bodybuilders are now regular guests on television talk shows. Always at the forefront of bodybuilding trends, Joe Weider turned a good part of *Muscle & Fitness* over to women's bodybuilding, and in 1981 he started *Shape,* a magazine devoted entirely to women. What's more, women's contests are staged in prestige settings like Atlantic City and Las Vegas, and beamed around the world on TV sports shows.

When the book *Pumping Iron* hit the newsstands in 1974 it contained not one word about women bodybuilders. The 1981 revised and updated edition, however, has a whole chapter on the female branch of the sport. The 1980 Miss Olympia, Rachel McLish, and company are featured right alongside the men.

Yes, women's bodybuilding has arrived. Women have brought a new dimension to the sport, a new vitality. They've put bodybuilding in the public eye like never before. Women are indeed a serious, and welcome, part of bodybuilding.

Due to the hormonal differences, a female bodybuilder can't develop muscles like a male bodybuilder. That's because the average woman has far fewer muscle-building hormones (androgenic hormones) than a man.

What women bodybuilders do develop is a trim, firm, feminine physique. Women who train with weights have more curves than women who don't. Women who take up weight training have everything to gain: firm arms, shapely legs, trim midsection and curvaceous hips. Bodybuilding gives women control over their bodies. Yes, it's easy to understand why women are serious about bodybuilding.

The diet and training information in this book applies to women as well as men. Actually, sensible diet and exercise are even more important for women. Women have less muscle mass then men and it's harder for them to build muscles. Women can't afford to sacrifice muscle in order to lose fat. Extreme diets and overtraining are damaging to the male physique, but they're even worse for women. Loss of muscle tissue can make a woman's physique flat and stringy. On the other hand, lean muscle gives a woman curves and shapes. When women lose fat *and* gain muscle tissue, the feminine physique truly emerges. Get ripped, ladies.

Youngsters

Lifting weights is one of the most positive things I did as a youth. I started training off and on when I was about 12, and by age 14 I

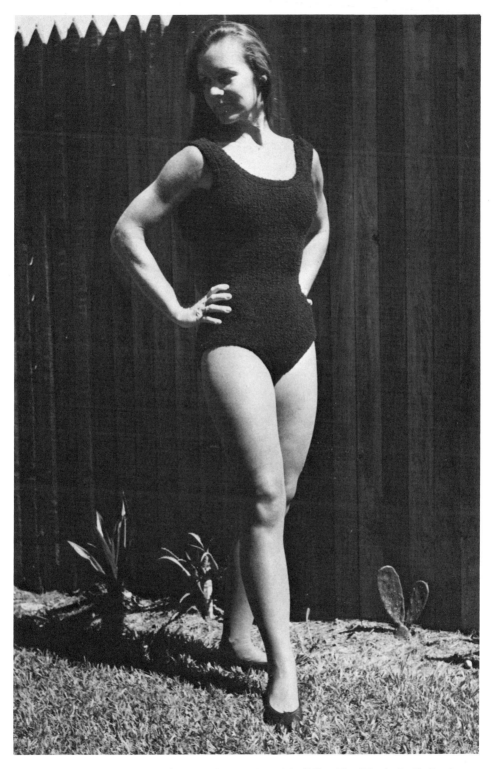

Vera Christensen is one of the pioneers of women's bodybuilding. Her "To the Ladies" column has appeared in *Strength & Health* magazine continuously since 1956. *Photo courtesy of Vera Christensen.*

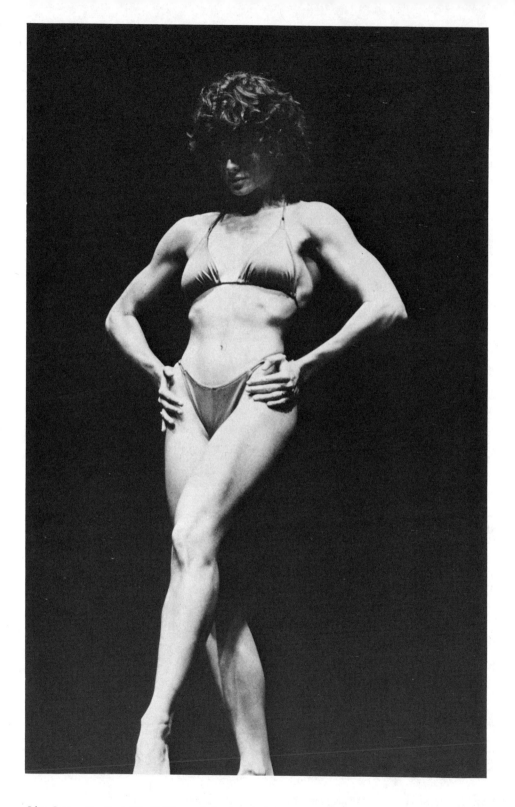

Lisa Lyon, the first World Woman's Bodybuilding Champion. *Photo courtesy of Muscle & Fitness magazine.*

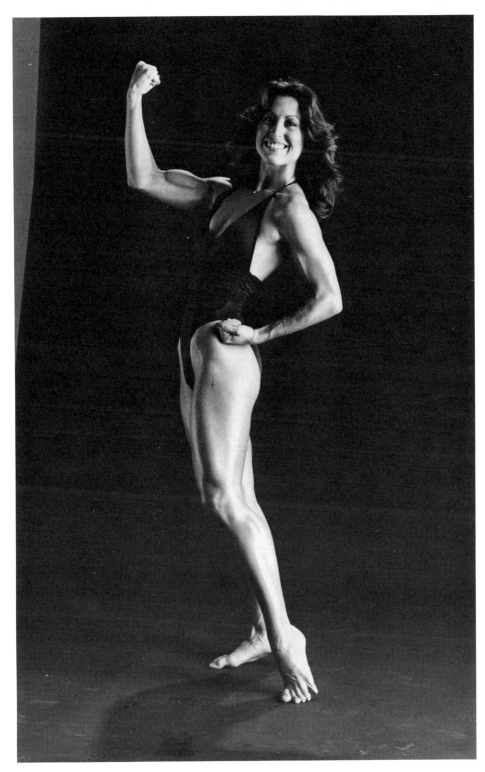

In 1980 Rachel McLish won the women's top professional title, Miss Olympia. She placed 2nd in 1981 and she's one of the favorites to win the title in 1982. *Photo courtesy of Muscle & Fitness magazine.*

was training regularly. Weight training taught me early that working at something conscientiously pays dividends. The habits I developed in weightlifting—especially consistency—carried over into other areas of my life. They helped me in college and law school, and they help me now as a lawyer.

Discovering at an early age that I could lift more weight than most other boys gave me self-confidence. It enhanced my self-image and helped me weather my adolescent years. My high school principal said I came to his school with the reputation of a delinquent and graduated a model student. Lifting had a lot to do with my transformation. It made me feel good about myself.

My early exposure to weight training had the added bonus of making me aware of the importance of good diet. I grew up reading about protein and vitamins. When my contemporaries were reading comic books, I was reading Bob Hoffman's articles on nutrition in *Strength & Health* magazine. As a teenager I became convinced of the evils of what Bob Hoffman called "the jitterbug diet." I would never even consider skipping breakfast or making a lunch out of Coke and chips. I bought so much Hoffman's Hi-Proteen Powder that the health food store gave me a discount.

My parents never had to get on me about my nutritional habits. Weightlifting motivated me to eat good food in a way that no amount of nagging from my parents could have done. I hope I can find a similar way to make my son aware of the importance of diet and nutrition. Most of us know what to tell our children about food, but the trick is to make them want to follow our advice. Getting kids involved in bodybuilding is the best way I know to instill sound nutritional habits.

Another advantage to getting youngsters involved in weight training is that it makes them less likely to become fat. Exercise burns calories and it also stabilizes the appetite. As previously mentioned, the adolescent growth spurt is one of the three periods when the number of fat cells can increase significantly in the body. Kids that exercise and eat right probably won't become fat adults. Weight training and a good diet kept me lean as a teenager and laid the groundwork for me to become a lean adult.

The diet and training information in this book applies to youngsters as well as adults. It's important to remember, however, that kids, like adults, should work into weight training gradually. Young bodybuilders should pay particular attention to good form in all exercises. Kids under 14 don't need to be concerned about lifting heavy weights. They should concentrate on doing the exercises correctly and getting a feel for how their muscles work. Two or three full-body workouts a week is a good way for young bodybuilders to begin. They should stick to basic exercises and keep their workouts short. Most important of all, their training should be fun. There will be plenty of time later to push the poundages up, if that's what they want to do.

My father inspired and encouraged me to train with weights, but he never pushed me. He was a track-and-field champion during his schoolboy days. He excelled in the discus, broad jump, high jump and pole vault. He was practically a one-man track team. I wanted to follow in his footsteps. Mainly, I wanted to be "strong."

I started out with his weights. He let me use them, but he never insisted that I train. I lifted because I wanted to lift. The way he steered me into competitive lifting shows his low-key approach. He asked me if I would like to see a local contest. I wasn't too interested, so he didn't force the issue. He planted the seed in my mind and let it go at that. I continued to train and when the contest came around the next year I wasn't in the audience. Instead, I competed and won my first medal. My father handled my introduction to weight training with a perfect balance of encouragement and restraint. I hope I can do as well for my son.

Set a good example for your children, make training facilities available, offer advice and encouragement, but don't push. Pressuring kids to train is the surest way to turn them off to exercise. I remember being ordered to run and do Push-Ups when I was in the Air Force. Had that been my introduction to exercise, I probably wouldn't be writing this book today.

One of the most constructive things you can do for your children, boys and girls, is motivate them to exercise and eat sensibly. For youngsters, the key word is "encourage." Don't push. Don't pressure. Encourage.

My Training Routine

My training routine is constantly evolving. I try new exercises, drop others and revive still others. I'm always searching for a better way to train. Sometimes I change just for the sake of change. A new

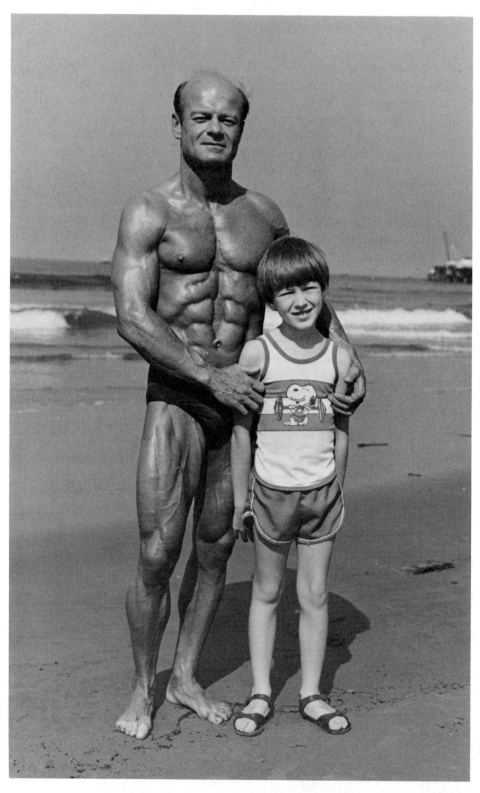

Matt Bass and friend. *Photo by Bill Reynolds.*

exercise or a new routine always gives me renewed enthusiasm ... training. Besides, it's good to work the muscles from many different angles.

So the routine I present here isn't exactly what I did a month ago and it's probably not what I'll be doing a month from now. Nevertheless, it's a good routine. It works for me and it will work for most bodybuilders.

That's not to suggest, however, that you should follow my routine blindly. Study what I do and pay special attention to how I've incorporated many of the training ideas presented in this book. Then adapt my routine to your own special circumstances. Remember Bill Dellinger's words: "The important thing is the principles of the program."

This is the type of routine I follow about six months out of the year. It's my normal non-peaking routine. During my three-month peaking period, I do fewer exercises and use high-intensity techniques such as negative and forced repetitions. For about three months after a peak, I do more exercise and use lighter weights.

Here's what I do on each of the four days of my training cycle:

DAY ONE
Upper back, Chest, Rear Deltoids and Upper Abdominals

Up at 4:00 a.m.
Record body weight and waist measurement
Light snack at 4:30
Workout at 5:00 (approximately one hour)

Workout
Brief General Warm-up: Overhead Arm Stretches, Toe Touch Stretches and Deep Knee Bends

UPPER BACK:

Nautilus Pullover:	1 set, 6-10 reps
Behind-Neck Lat Machine Pulldown:	1 set, 6-10 reps (shoulder width, palms facing grip)
One-Arm Dumbell Row:	1 set, 6-10 reps with each arm (use straps for grip)

103

| One-Arm Pulley Row: (see photos) | 1 set, 6-10 reps with each arm |

CHEST

| One-Arm Pec Deck: | 1 set, 6-10 reps with each arm (hold on with free arm) |

| Crossover Pulley for Upper Pecs: (see photo) | 1 set, 6-10 reps (bottom handles, standing jackknife position) |

| Crossover Pulley for Outer Pecs: (see photo) | 1 set, 6-10 reps (top handles, upright position) |

| Parallel Bar Dips | 1 set, 6-10 reps (head down, feet forward, elbows out, attach weight) |

I alternate upper back and chest exercises as follows: Pullover, Pec Deck, Pulldown, Crossover, Dumbbell Row, Crossover, Pulley Row and Dips. This allows better recuperation and greater effort on each upper back and chest exercise.

REAR DELTOIDS:

| Dumbbell Bentover Lateral Raise: | 1 set, 6-10 reps |

UPPER ABDOMINALS:

| Vertical Sit-Ups (see photo) | 1 set, 6-10 reps (hold dumbbell on chest) |

Walk:	6:30, approximately 3 miles
Breakfast:	7:30
Lunch:	12 Noon
Snack:	3:30
Stationary bicycle:	6:00 p.m. 30 minutes plus brief warm-up and warm down
Dinner:	7:00 p.m.
Light snack:	8:30
Bed:	9:00

DAY TWO
Lower Back, Calves, Thighs and Obliques

Up at 4:00 a.m.
Record body weight and waist measurement
Light snack at 4:30
Workout at 5:00 (approximately one hour)

Workout

Brief General Warm-up: Same as Day One

LOWER BACK:

Nautilus Hip & Back Machine: 1 set, 6-10 reps

Bent-Knee Deadlift: 1 set, 6-10 reps (Use straps for grip, do not allow back to become rounded, lift smoothly, use legs)

CALVES:

Standing Calf Raise
on Machine: 1 set, 6-10 reps

Seated Calf Raise
on Machine: 1 set, 6-10 reps

THIGHS:

Leg Extension: 1 set, 6-10 reps

Full Squat: 1 set, 6-10 reps (Heels elevated, upright position, keep back straight)

Leg Press: 1 set, 6-10 reps

Hack Squat: 1 set, 6-10 reps

Leg Curl: 1 set, 6-10 reps

OBLIQUES:

Dumbbell Side Bends: (see photo)	1 set, 6-10 reps each side (Use straps for grip.)
Twisting Pulldown: (see photo)	1 set, 6-10 reps to each side
Twisting Sit-Ups on Steep Incline:	1 set, 10-12 reps (5-6 each side)

The balance of my daily schedule is the same as Day One.

DAY THREE
Traps, Shoulders, Biceps, Triceps, Lower Abdominals

Up at 4:00 a.m.
Record body weight and waist measurement
Light snack at 4:30
Workout at 5:00 (approximately one hour)

Workout

Brief General Warm-Up:	Same as Day One

TRAPS:

Dumbbell Shrugs:	1 set, 6-10 reps (use straps for grip)

SHOULDERS:

One-Arm Dumbbell Side Lateral Raise:	1 set, 6-10 reps with each arm (support yourself with free arm)
Standing Barbell Press:	1 set, 6-10 reps
Pulley Upright Row:	1 set, 6-10 reps (shoulder-width grip)

BICEPS:

Two-Arm Curl on Nautilus Multi-Biceps Machine:	1 set, 6-10 reps
Dumbbell Curl on Incline Bench:	1 set, 6-10 reps

One-Arm Preacher Bench Curl
(45° angle) from Low Pulley: 1 set, 6-10 reps with each arm

Narrow-Grip Curl on E-Z
Curl Bar: 1 set, 6-10 reps

TRICEPS

Triceps Pushdown on   1 set, 6-10 reps
Lat Machine: (narrow grip with V-handle)

Triceps Pushdown on   1 set, 6-10 reps (shoulder-width
Lat Machine: grip with straight bar)

Two-Arm Dumbbell Kickback
on Incline Bench: 1 set, 6-10 reps
(see photo)

Close Grip Bench Press
with E-Z Curl Bar: 1 set, 6-10 reps

LOWER ABDOMINALS:

Hip Curl-Up on Sit-Up   1 set, up to 30 reps
Board (see photos)

The balance of my daily schedule is the same as Day One.

DAY FOUR
Rest Day

Up at approximately 5:30 a.m.
Record body weight and waist measurement
Light snack at 6:00
Walk or outdoor bike ride at 6:30 (approximately one hour)

The balance of my schedule is the same as Day One, except I don't
ride the stationary bicycle before dinner.

SOME EXPLANATION

WARM-UP: My general warm-up at the beginning of each workout is designed to get the blood flowing, help me wake up and put me in the mood to train. It's very brief—5-6 overhead arm stretches, 5-6 toe touch stretches and about 10 deep knee bends—but it helps!

I also do a specific warm-up for each exercise. For big muscle groups, like the back and legs, I do two or three warm-up sets. For smaller groups, like the shoulders and arms, I do one or two warm-up sets. I use a weight considerably below the weight I plan to use for my maximum set, and I only do enough repetitions to warm up. For example, if I plan to squat with 300 pounds for eight reps on my heavy set, I might do the following warm-up sets: 135 x 5, 205 x 3, 255 x 3.

Warming up increases the elasticity of the tendons and ligaments and causes a rise in the temperature of the muscle cells. It's a safeguard against injury. A cold muscle simply isn't prepared to perform up to capacity. A warm-up is important, but it shouldn't tire you out. Warm up, but don't overdo it. Save your energy for the sets that count, the heavy sets.

EXERCISE SELECTION: I choose up to four exercises for each body part. I do more exercises for complex muscles, like the chest and upper back, than for simple muscles, like calves and traps. The latissimus (upper back) and pectorals (chest) are big muscles capable of a variety of movements, while the calves and traps are smaller and perform in a more limited range. Simple muscles can be worked through their full range of motion with only one or two exercises. It takes more exercises to fully activate complex muscles. I work each muscle from several different angles to stimulate all the muscle fibers, and try to work every muscle through its full range of motion.

In any routine I'm careful to work the upper and lower lats, the upper, middle and lower pecs, upper and lower biceps, the long and short heads of the triceps, the front, side and rear deltoids, the upper and lower quadriceps, and both the soleus and gastrocnemius of the calf muscles. On some muscles like the quadriceps I probably do more exercises than necessary. I enjoy working my quads.

I think it's important to include the Squat and Deadlift in most routines because of their overall body stimulating effect. Simply put, they're two of the best exercises you can do. They stimulate overall growth, increase endurance and build great strength.

TRAINING CYCLES: I use the hard-day, easy-day principle discussed earlier. I vary the intensity of my workouts over four training cycles, or 16 days. During this period I train my body heavy (100%) twice, medium (85%) once, and light (70%) once. My first four-day training cycle is 100 percent, my second 85 percent, my third 100 percent and my fourth 70 percent. In short, my training cycle is: heavy, medium, heavy and light. I follow every heavy cycle with a medium or light cycle.

I use the heaviest weight I can on my heavy cycles. I use less weight on my medium and light cycles. For example, on the Nautilus Leg Extension I'm currently using the whole weight stack, 24 plates, for six reps during my heavy cycle. On the medium cycle (85%) I do six reps with 20 plates and on my light cycle (70%) I use 17 plates for six reps. I calculate my poundages before each workout on the basis of the weight I used during my last heavy cycle. I spend a few minutes with a calculator figuring my poundages before each workout.

The heavy-medium-heavy-light poundage variation is probably the most important feature of my training routine. Most bodybuilders don't vary the intensity of their workouts, but I'm convinced they should. Medium and light cycles allow full recovery from heavy cycles. Remember, there can be no growth without adequate rest and recovery. The harder you train, the more you must rest.

EXERCISE FORM: Progression is the essence of bodybuilding. To make gains you must lift heavier and heavier weights. But don't cheat in order to raise the weight. Don't sacrifice form. Sometimes I get ahead of myself. I find myself doing shorter or faster reps so I can lift more. When this happens I lower the weight and make a special effort to do slow, controlled, full-range repetitions. To remind myself, I write it in my training diary: "Do slow, controlled, full reps." I'm usually surprised how much more I feel the muscle action when I lower the weight and do it right. It's safer, too.

Advice for Beginners

Most beginners have what I call a "virgin body." That's a great advantage, because it means they'll grow stronger and bigger on a very simple routine. A beginner's body isn't used to the stress of weight training and, therefore, responds readily to minimum stimulation. A beginner is also less able to make inroads into his or her recovery capacity and, therefore, recuperates from workouts quickly. Most beginners don't need to vary the intensity of their workouts; they can train hard every workout. Here's a good basic routine for beginners:

1) General Warm-up:

Overhead Arm Stretch	10 reps
Side Bend	10 reps
Toe Touch	10 reps
Deep Knee Bend	10 reps
2) Full Squat*	two sets of 10 reps
3) Bent-Knee Deadlift*	two sets of 10 reps
4) Standing Toe Raise*	two sets of 10 reps
5) Barbell Bentover Row	two sets of 10 reps
6) Bench Press*	two sets of 10 reps
7) Standing Press	two sets of 10 reps
8) Barbell Curl*	two sets of 10 reps
9) Lying Triceps Extension*	two sets of 10 reps
10) Bent-Knee Sit-Ups*	two sets of 10 reps or until abdominal muscles are fatigued

*Do one or two warm-up sets of 5-6 reps with light to medium weight.

A beginner should start out conservatively. If you have any health problems or if you are over 40, consult your physician before starting on a weight training program. Use your first few workouts as a break-in period. Train with light weights and learn how to do each exercise properly. After a one- or two-week break-in period, a beginner should start training three times a week, with at least one rest day between sessions. On each exercise select a weight that makes the last rep or two hard. Do slow, controlled, full-range reps. Again, don't sacrifice form to lift heavier weights. Don't do more sets than suggested. If you're not recovering between workouts, drop one set of each exercise.

It's beyond the scope of this book to explain how to perform basic exercise. Bill Pearl's book *Keys to the Inner Universe** has the most complete list of exercises ever assembled. Each exercise is

110

clearly explained with drawings and text. Pearl's book also offers typical routines for beginning, intermediate and advanced bodybuilders.

In addition, any large bookstore will have a number of bodybuilding books which explain the basic exercises and provide beginner, intermediate and advanced routines.** You may also want to consider going to a gym or health club. If you decide to go this route, I suggest that you ask around and find out where the competitive bodybuilders in your area train. That's the place to go for sound instruction.

Keys to the Inner Universe is available from Bill Pearl, 100 South Michigan Avenue, P.O. Box 4625, Pasadena, CA 91106 (Price $32.95 plus 10% postage). Ripped Enterprises also carries this book.

**Joe Weider's book, *Bodybuilding: The Weider Approach* (Contemporary Books, Inc. 1981) has a fully annotated bibliography of the currently available books.

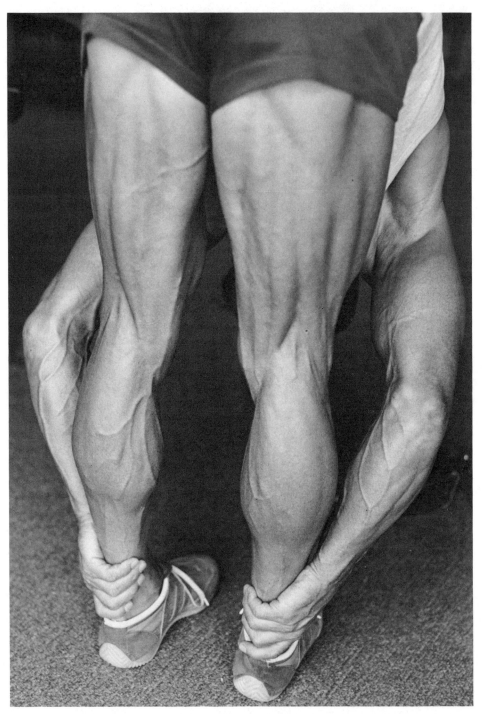

The Toe Touch Stretch is part of my general warm-up. *Photo by Bill Reynolds.*

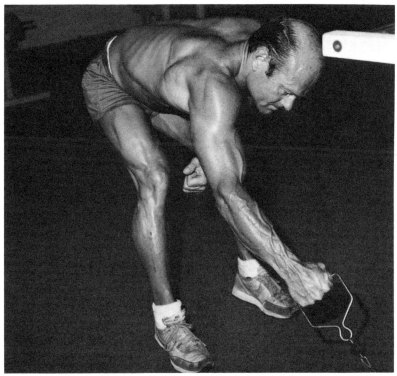

Start of One-Arm Pulley Row.

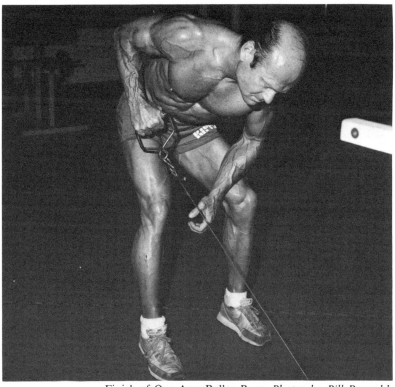

Finish of One-Arm Pulley Row. *Photos by Bill Reynolds.*

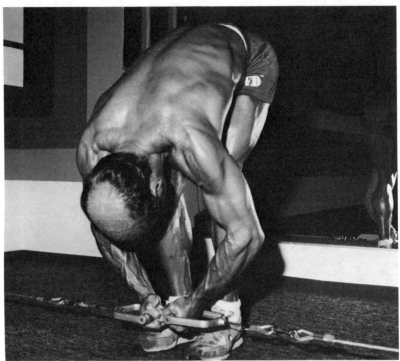

Crossover Pulley for Upper Pecs. *Photo by Bill Reynolds.*

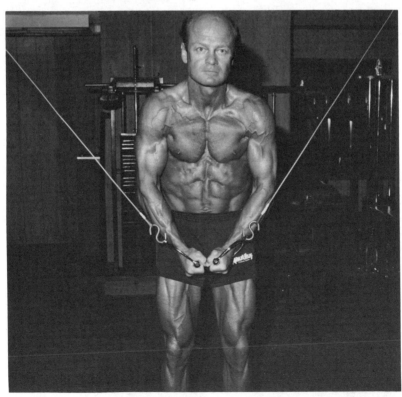

Crossover Pulley for Outer Pecs. *Photo by Bill Reynolds.*

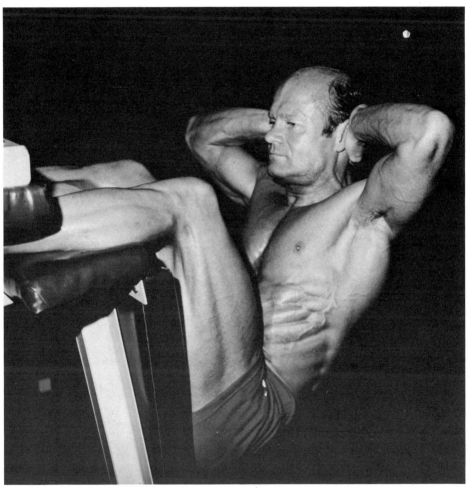

Vertical Sit-Up for Upper Abs. *Photo by Bill Reynolds.*

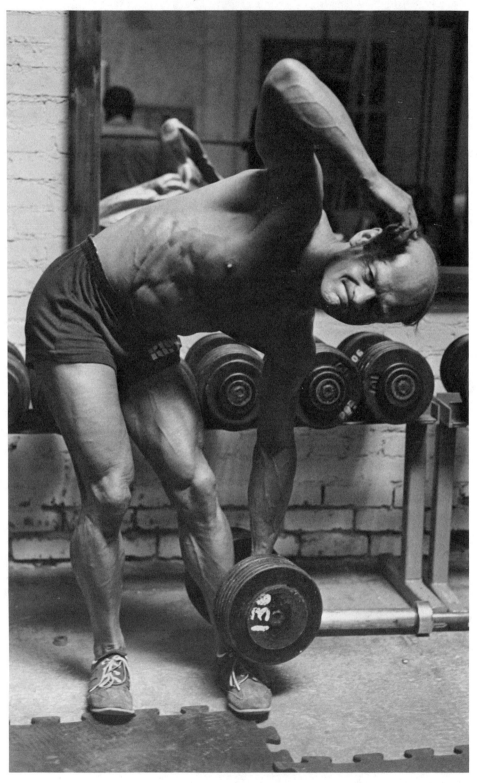

Dumbbell Side Bend. *Photo by Bill Reynolds.*

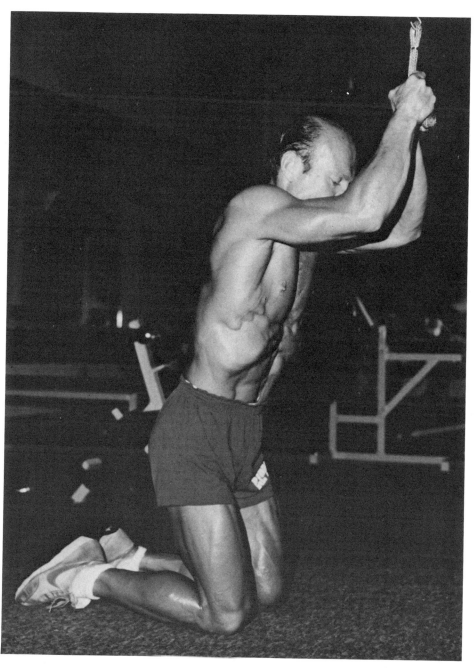

Twisting Pulldown. Pulldown like you're bowing. Alternate from side to side bringing elbows across body and down by the opposite knee. *Photo by Bill Reynolds.*

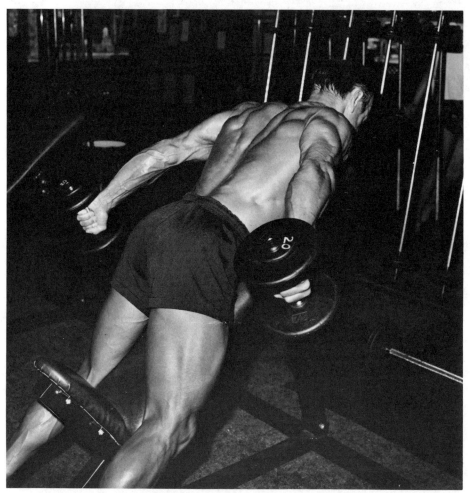

Two-Arm Dumbbell Kickback on Incline Bench. *Photo by Bill Reynolds.*

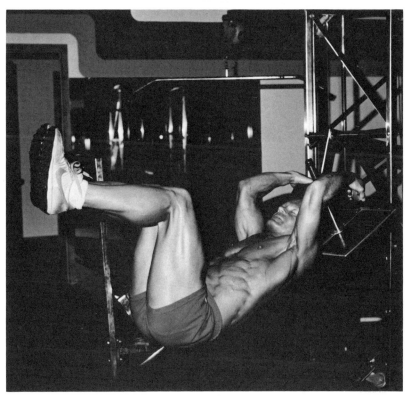

Start of Hip Curl-Up on Sit-Up Board. *Photo by Bill Reynolds.*

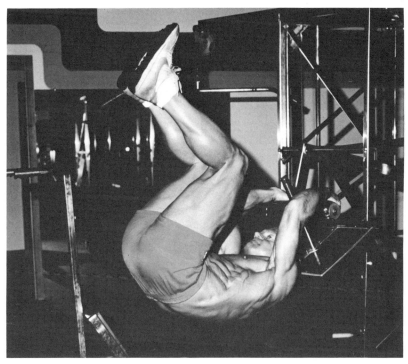

Finish of Hip Curl-Up on Sit-Up Board. *Photo by Bill Reynolds.*

"It takes only one properly placed shot to kill a rabbit, or an elephant. Additional shots will serve no purpose except unnecessary destruction of the meat. The same is true of exercise."
—Arthur Jones, Inventor of Nautilus machines.

PART THREE

Peaking

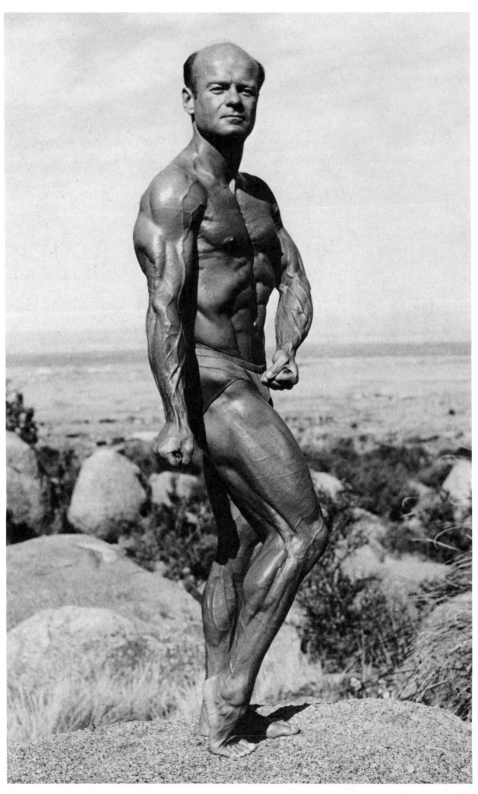

Photo by Allen Hughes.

PART III: PEAKING

The Final Push

Conventional bodybuilding wisdom has it—erroneously—that the way to get into contest shape is to train lighter and longer. The idea seems to be that training lighter and longer will make a bodybuilder more muscular, more defined, because it burns the fat off. To some extent it does, but it's not the best or most effective way to reduce body fat.

What a bodybuilder wants on the day of the contest is minimum fat *and* maximum muscle. Diet and aerobic exercise are the best ways to lose fat, and high-intensity weight training is the best way to build and retain muscle. But training lighter and longer means using fewer muscle fibers. And muscle fibers that aren't being used will probably be lost (the "use-it-or-lose-it" principle comes into play). So training lighter and longer results in loss of muscle, which certainly isn't what you want.

To develop maximum muscle at contest time, you must train harder and less. Bodybuilders can learn from runners when it comes to achieving contest condition. The goal of the runner and the bodybuilder is much the same. Both strive to bring their muscles to a physiological peak for competition.

In his *Guide for the Elite Runner,* Marty Liquori tells how runners peak for competition. In the last few weeks before the big race, they rest more. They drop mileage so they can increase intensity. Liquori explains: "The workouts themselves... will be faster (and) more condensed. ...Instead of 12 x 400 in 62, the elite runner will now try to do 6 in 57." In short, runners get the most out of themselves by training harder and less.

Repeatedly, I've achieved my best condition by training harder and less. In 1979 I hit 2.4 percent body fat twice, while gaining muscle at the same time (see graph five on page 76 of *Ripped*). In May 1980 and August 1981, I reduced to 3.1 percent and 2.7 percent body fat, respectively, while gaining muscle (see graph three and four). Each time my workouts were short and heavy.

The last month or two before a contest a bodybuilder should train less so he or she can train harder. That's what I did during the months of June and July in 1981, when I increased my lean body weight from 147.9 to 163.1 pounds and reduced my body fat from 5.2 percent to 2.7 percent. During that two-month period, I gained 15.2 pounds of muscle and lost 3.6 pounds of fat (see graph four).

On heavy days during that period I intensified my workouts by cutting my exercises in half. For example, I reduced my upper back exercises from four to two. I didn't increase my sets. After a warm-up, I did *one* super hard set of each exercise. Previously, I'd been doing Pullovers, Pulldowns, Pulley Rows and Dumbbell Rows. When I started my peaking period. I did only two of those exercises in each workout. I would do Pullovers and Dumbbell Rows one session and Pulldowns and Pulley Rows the next. I used rest-pause, force reps, negatives or negative-accentuated reps on almost every exercise. I made similar adjustments for other body parts. I trained less, I trained harder, and I gained muscle and lost fat.

In 1981, when I shifted gears and started pushing towards a peak, I knew that I was training over my head, that I was getting ahead of myself. I knew I was heading for a sticking point. The trick is to time your peak so you play out your string and hit the sticking point at contest time—not before. This takes practice.

The "coaxing gains" method that I mentioned earlier should be used during the first part of the peaking period. Keep everything under control. Do your reps slowly, contract hard at the end of each

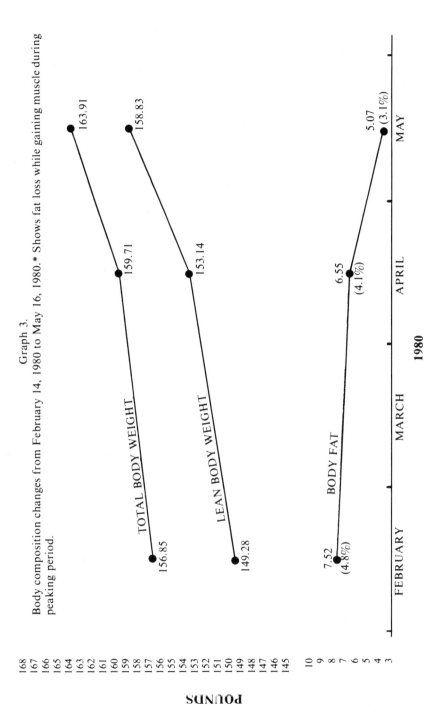

Graph 3.

Body composition changes from February 14, 1980 to May 16, 1980.* Shows fat loss while gaining muscle during peaking period.

TOTAL BODY WEIGHT

163.91
159.71
156.85

LEAN BODY WEIGHT

158.83
153.14
149.28

BODY FAT

7.52
(4.8%)
6.55
(4.1%)
5.07
(3.1%)

1980

FEBRUARY   MARCH   APRIL   MAY

POUNDS

168
167
166
165
164
163
162
161
160
159
158
157
156
155
154
153
152
151
150
149
148
147
146
145

10
9
8
7
6
5
4
3

*Body composition tests performed by Lovelace Medical Center, Research Division, Albuquerque, New Mexico.

POUNDS

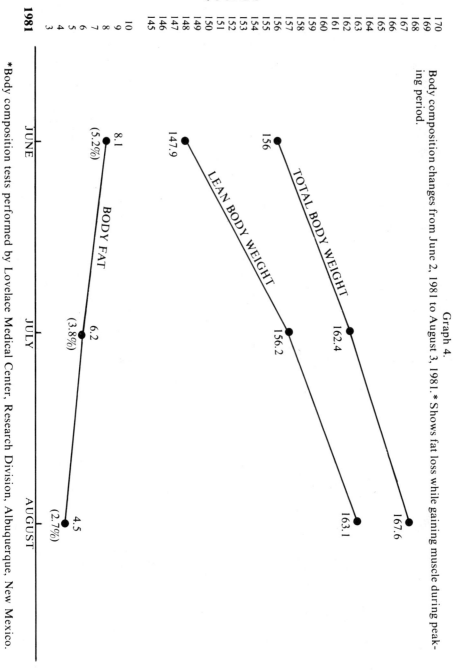

Graph 4.
Body composition changes from June 2, 1981 to August 3, 1981.* Shows fat loss while gaining muscle during peaking period.

*Body composition tests performed by Lovelace Medical Center, Research Division, Albuquerque, New Mexico.

rep and stop your set just short of your absolute limit. Stop at a point which gives you confidence you can do a little more next time.

It's only at the very end of the peaking phase, the last two or three weeks, that you should push to your absolute limit. At that point, you're after maximum possible muscle gains over the short term. The fact that you can't keep it up for long is of no concern. You want as much muscle as possible at contest time. You're not concerned about hitting a sticking point after the contest. You know you'll have to take a rest then anyway. So you pull out all the stops. As Marty Liquori puts it, "This is the time to go to the afterburners."

When you pull out the stops, however, you do so advisedly. You know you're stepping over the line. You know you're coming to the top of the hill and that you'll probably stumble over the top and take a dive. That's what peaking is all about. You peak, and then you take it easy for a while. You plan it that way.

During my peaking period in 1981, I used forced reps, negatives and rest-pause during heavy cycles only. I thought I was allowing myself to recuperate by training in regular style every other cycle. I lowered my poundages and—here's the problem—did more reps. I did as many reps as I could even on my "light" cycles. In effect, I trained heavy every workout, which was a mistake. When I increased my intensity, I should have increased my rest as well. Next time I go for a peak, I'll follow every high-intensity cycle with a light cycle, about 75 percent with no increase in sets or reps.

Brooks Johnson, head track coach at Stanford University, summed it up in an article on peaking in *Runner's World* magazine: "As the intensity of training increases, there must be commensurate increase in the rest and recovery periods." Remember, pre-contest training for a bodybuilder should be heavier and shorter. You must train less so you can train harder.

I'll close this section with a few words of caution: unless you're preparing for competition, you probably won't want to engage in the type of peaking training I've just described. You're more interested in steady, continuous gains. You have no reason to try and get ahead of yourself. However, if you do decide to train for a peak, realize you'll have to relax afterwards. Then you'll need to build up again. Enjoy the peak, but be prepared for the valley. As long as your peaks keep getting higher, you're doing all right.

Finally, be careful. High-intensity training can lead to injury.

Don't use loose form so you can lift more weight. Slow, controlled reps are best, whether you're peaking or not. Good form produces better results, and you experience fewer injuries.

Here's an example of a peaking routine:

DAY ONE
Upper Back, Chest, Rear Delts and Upper Abs

GENERAL WARM-UP: Same as before.

UPPER BACK:

Nautilus Pullover:	1 set rest-pause style, 5 + 3 + 2 reps 1 set negative-accentuated style, 4-6 reps with each arm (lift with both arms and lower with one arm; do each arm separately; weight approximately 70% of regular style)
Behind-Neck Lat Machine Pulldown:	1 set, 4-6 reps plus 2-3 forced reps plus 2-3 negative reps (medium width, palms facing grip)
One-Arm Dumbbell Row:	1 set rest-pause style, 5 + 3 + 2 reps with each arm (use straps for grip)

CHEST:

One-Arm Pec Deck:	1 set rest-pause style, 5 + 3 + 2 reps with each arm
Incline Bench Press on Universal-Type Machine:	1 set rest-pause style, 5 + 3 + 2 reps
Parallel Bar Dips:	1 set rest-pause style, 5 + 3 + 2 reps (attach weight; head down, feet forward, elbows out)

REAR DELTS:

Dumbbell Bentover Lateral Raise:	1 set rest-pause style, 5 + 3 + 2 reps

UPPER ABS:

Vertical Sit-Ups:

1 set, 6-8 reps plus 2-4 negative reps (dumbbell on chest; for negative reps use arms to raise weight to top position)

DAY TWO
Traps, Lower Back, Calves, Thighs and Obliques

GENERAL WARM-UP: Same

TRAPS:

Barbell Shrugs:

1 set rest-pause style, 5 + 3 + 2 reps (use straps for grip)

LOWER BACK:

Bent-Knee Deadlift:

1 set, 6-8 reps (use your legs; do not allow back to become rounded; use straps for grips)

CALVES:

Standing Calf Raise: 1 set rest-pause style, 5 + 3 + 2 reps

Seated Calf Raise: 1 set rest-pause style, 5 + 3 + 2 reps

THIGHS:

Leg Extension:

1 set rest-pause style, 5 + 3 + 2 reps 1 set negative-accentuated style, 4-6 reps with each leg (raise with both legs, lower with one leg; do each leg separately; weight approximately 70% of regular style)

Leg Press: 1 set rest-pause style, 5 + 3 + 2 reps

Hack Squat: 1 set rest-pause style, 5 + 3 + 2 reps

Leg Curl:	1 set rest-pause style, 5 + 3 + 2 reps 1 set negative-accentuated style, 4-6 reps with each leg (lift with both legs, lower with one leg; do each leg separately; weight approximately 70-80% of regular style)

OBLIQUES:

Dumbbell Side Bend:	1 set, 6-10 reps for each side (use straps for grip)

DAY THREE
Shoulders, Biceps, Triceps and Lower Abs

GENERAL WARM-UP:	Same

SHOULDERS:

One-Arm Dumbbell Side Lateral Raise:	1 set rest-pause style, 5 + 3 + 2 reps with each arm (brace yourself with free arm)
Seated Press on Universal- Type Machine:	1 set rest-pause style, 5 + 3 + 2 reps

BICEPS:

Two-Arm Curl on Biceps Machine:	1 set rest-pause style, 5 + 3 + 2 reps
One-Arm Preacher Bench Curl (45° angle) from Low Pulley:	1 set rest-pause style, 5 + 3 + 2 reps with each arm
One-Arm Negative Dumbbell Curls on Preacher Bench (90° angle):	1 set negative-style only, 6-8 reps with each arm (raise dumbbell with both arms or have training partner help)

TRICEPS:

Triceps Pushdown on Lat Machine:	1 set, 4-6 reps plus 3-4 negative reps (straight bar, medium grip; have training partner help on negative reps)
One-Arm Dumbbell Kickbacks:	1 set rest-pause style, 5 + 3 + 2 reps with each arm
Close-Grip Reverse Triceps Extension on Flat Bench with E-Z Curl Bar:	1 set, 6-8 reps, (press weight up and lower as in Triceps Extension)

LOWER ABS:

Hip Curl-up on Sit-Up Board (see photo in Part Two)	1 set rest-pause style, 15 + 10 + 8 reps or until lower abs tired before each pause

DAY FOUR
Rest Day

COMMENTS

Do a specific warm-up for each exercise, but don't overdo it.

Follow each heavy cycle with a light cycle (75%). On the light cycles, do one set (6-10 reps) on each exercise in regular style, using about 75 percent of maximum weight. For example, if your maximum for 10 reps is 100 pounds, then do 10 reps with 75 pounds.

Aerobic exercise—walking, biking, etc.—should be continued during the peaking period to facilitate recovery between workouts and to burn off fat.

The workouts in this peaking routine are short to allow maximum effort on each and every exercise. Make every set count. Remember to do slow, controlled, full reps. I begin my peaking routine with poundages I can handle in absolutely strict form. It's important to start off on a positive note. Do each exercise hard, but with precision.

It's OK to adapt this routine to your needs. But keep the principle of a peaking routine in mind: train less, so you can train harder.

Now here's an example of a general conditioning routine for the "down" period after a peak:

DAY ONE
Upper Back, Chest and Upper Abs

GENERAL WARM-UP:	Same as before

UPPER BACK:

Wide-Grip Front Lat Machine Pulldown:	1 set, 10 reps
Barbell Bentover Row:	1 set, 10 reps
Medium-Reverse-Grip Front Lat Machine Pulldown:	1 set, 10 reps
T-Bar Row:	1 set, 10 reps
Narrow-Grip V-Bar Lat Machine Pulldown:	1 set, 10 reps
Seated One-Arm Row from High Pulley:	1 set, 10 reps with each arm
Wide-Grip Lat Machine Pulldown with Body Back at 45° Angle:	1 set, 10 reps

CHEST:

Crossover Pulley for Middle Pec (see photo):	1 set, 10 reps (top pulley; bend over at 90°)
Dumbbell Bench Press:	1 set, 10 reps
Incline Bench Fly from Low Pulleys:	1 set, 10 reps
Incline Bench Dumbbell Press:	1 set, 10 reps

Crossover Pulley for Lower Pec (see photo):	1 set, 10 reps (kneeling upright position from low pulleys)
Wide-Grip Dips:	1 set, 10 reps
Decline Bench Press:	1 set, 10 reps

UPPER ABS:

| Bent-Knee Sit-Ups: | 1 set, up to 20 reps |
| Crunches with Feet on Bench: | 1 set, up to 20 reps |

DAY TWO
Traps, Lower Back, Calves, Thighs, Obliques

| GENERAL WARM-UP: | Same as before |

TRAPS:

| Dumbbell Shrugs: | 1 set, 10 reps |

LOWER BACK:

| Stiff-Leg Deadlift: | 1 set, 10 reps |
| Bent-Knee Deadlift: | 1 set, 10 reps |

CALVES:

Toe Press on Leg Press Machine:	1 set, 10 reps
One-Leg Standing Calf Raise:	1 set, 10 reps with each leg
Seated Calf Raise:	1 set, 10 reps

THIGHS:

Leg Extension:	1 set, 10 reps
Flat-Footed Squat with Medium Foot Spacing:	1 set, 10 reps
Flat-Footed Squat with Wide Foot Spacing:	1 set, 10 reps

Heels-Elevated Squat with Narrow Foot Spacing:	1 set, 10 reps
Leg Press with Medium Foot Spacing:	1 set, 10 reps
Leg Press with Narrow Foot Spacing:	1 set, 10 reps
Leg Curl:	3 sets, 10 reps

OBLIQUES:

Dumbbell Side Bend:	1 set, 10 reps each side
Twisting Bent-Knee Sit-Up On Steep Incline:	1 set, up to 20 reps
Twisting Pulldown from High Pulley: (see photo in Part Two)	1 set, 10 reps each side (kneeling position)

DAY THREE
Shoulders, Biceps, Triceps and Lower Abs

GENERAL WARM-UP:	Same as before

SHOULDERS:

One-Arm Side Lateral from Low Pulley:	1 set, 10 reps each arm
Alternate Dumbbell Press:	1 set, 10 reps
Narrow-Grip Barbell Upright Row:	1 set, 10 reps
Seated Press Behind Neck:	1 set, 10 reps
Wide-Grip Barbell Upright Row:	1 set, 10 reps
Dumbbell Front Lateral Raise:	1 set, 10 reps

BICEPS:

Seated Dumbbell Curl:	1 set, 10 reps
Incline-Bench Outward Dumb-bell Curl (curl in line with body):	1 set, 10 reps
Narrow-Grip E-Z Curl Bar Curl:	1 set, 10 reps
Lying-Flat Bench Curl from High Pulley (elbows up at 90° to body):	1 set, 10 reps
Kneeling Two-Arm Curl Behind Neck from High Pulley:	1 set, 10 reps

TRICEPS:

Dumbbell Triceps Extension on Flat Bench:	1 set, 10 reps
Kneeling Behind-Neck Triceps Extension from Low Pulley:	1 set, 10 reps
Wide-Grip Triceps Pushdown on Lat Machine:	1 set, 10 reps
Kneeling Bentover Dumbbell Kickbacks:	1 set, 10 reps
Dips:	1 set, 10 reps (head and feet back, elbows straight back)
Narrow-Grip Bench Press:	1 set, 10 reps

LOWER ABS:

Chinning-Bar Leg Raise:	1 set, reps until abs fatigued
Dip-Stand Leg Raise:	1 set, reps until abs fatigued
Leg Raise Sitting on End of Bench:	1 set, reps until abs fatigued

DAY FOUR
Rest Day

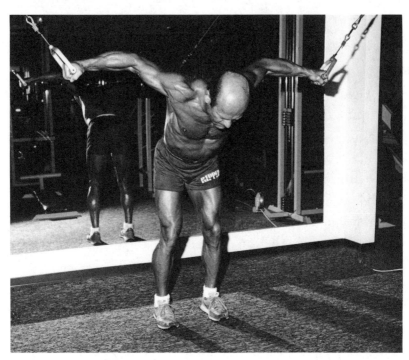

Crossover Pulley for Middle Pecs. *Photo by Bill Reynolds.*

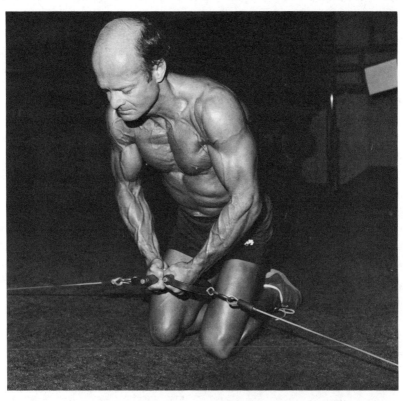

Crossover Pulley for Lower Pecs. *Photo by Bill Reynolds.*

COMMENTS

This high-volume routine is suitable for the period after a peak. Don't push during this period. Stick to light weights (about 75 percent of maximum). After a peak it's time to have fun with a wide variety of exercises you don't normally do. I use Bill Pearl's book, *Keys to the Inner Universe,* to help me select exercises that will work my muscles from many different angles. During this period I also ride my bike a lot to improve my aerobic fitness. This training phase should last 2-3 months in the yearly cycle.

A high-volume, low-intensity routine like this gets you in shape to train hard again later. Don't skip the general conditioning phase of training. It's an essential part of the yearly cycle. It recharges your battery and lays the groundwork for the coming season.

I divide my yearly training cycle more or less as follows:

3 months: high-volume, low-intensity.

6 months: medium-volume, medium-intensity.

3 months: low-volume, high-intensity.

The Famine Phenomenon

Incredible as it may seem, starving yourself before a contest can make you fatter. Cutting off the food supply shocks the body. Your body doesn't know you're preparing for a contest. It thinks a famine is coming, and it braces for the famine by storing extra fat to live on.

Our ancestors were often forced to go for days without food. They endured these short famines by living off stored fat. The ones who survived were those with the ability to store fat easily. They passed on that ability to us. We still store fat as a protective mechanism. We deposit a few calories out of each meal as fat to guard against possible famine. We respond to the stress of food restriction by conserving fat, by depositing it even though we're losing weight.

Covert Bailey, in his excellent book *Fit or Fat?*, says that "fasting will encourage your body to become fatter." He explains that research has proven that severe diets cause the body to produce more of the enzymes responsible for the depositing of fat. These fat-depositing enzymes create what he calls "a fat person's chemistry." They create a tendency to get fat.

137

Bailey explains the famine phenomenon like this: "Now if you can visualize that fat represents a magnificent safety device against famine, you can appreciate that the body will attempt to make more of it under stress circumstances. Temporary fasting is a stress.... Likewise, most diets that are high in protein and low in carbohydrate are translated as an emergency situation, bringing an increase in the depositing of fat."

Frankly, I didn't believe I could eat less and gain fat—until it happened to me... twice!

The TV program *PM Magazine* was doing a segment on my preparation for the 1980 Past-40 Mr. America contest. My last body composition test before the contest was going to be filmed for the program, and I wanted to be leaner than ever before—below 2.4 percent. A week earlier Lovelace Medical Center had measured my body fat at 3.1 percent, so I didn't have far to go. I was carrying 5.03 pounds of fat. I calculated that losing 1½ pounds of fat would bring me down to 2.2 percent body fat. Since 1½ pounds of fat contains 5,250 calories, simple division told me that I needed to reduce my calorie intake by 750 per day. I made the necessary adjustments in my diet and arrived for the test confident that I was ready for the TV cameras to film a new personal record for leanness.

When the procedure was completed, I sat before the cameras and waited for Dr. Michael D. Venters to complete his calculations. He signalled to the *PM Magazine* director that he was ready. The camera zoomed in to catch my expression when I heard the result. 3.7 percent! I couldn't faint before a national television audience, so I mumbled something about expecting to be a little lower. Actually, I couldn't believe I'd gained almost a pound of fat. It was mathematically impossible. I didn't known what to make of it. I wrote in my diary that Dr. Venters may have been unnerved by the cameras, causing him to misread the scales or make an error in his calculations. I also wrote that it was possible I had pushed by diet too hard.

Later that year I attended a seminar Covert Bailey presented to a group of dentists in Albuquerque. I perked up when he told the audience that rapid weight loss can cause an increase in fat storage. That evening I reread the detailed explanation in his book. But I guess I still didn't believe it, because I made the same mistake in 1981.

On August 21, 1981 I again equalled my record for leanness: 2.4 percent body fat. I decided to be weighed again in one week and go for a new record low.

It was a busy seven days. I kept my calories low, I trained, and I practiced my posing every day. I pedaled to exhaustion on the stationary bicycle at Lovelace Medical Center to measure my oxygen uptake capacity. I had two days of photo sessions with Bill Reynolds, the Editor-in-Chief of *Muscle & Fitness* magazine. I was sure I'd burned up enough fat to go below 2.4 percent.

It was a disaster! I lost 5.6 pounds in seven days, but my body fat went *up* to 3.1 percent. I had lost 6.12 pounds of muscle, and I gained 1.06 pounds of fat. So I had done it again! I cut my calories too much. My body responded to the stress by depositing more fat, even though I was losing weight.

In the future I'm going to do my best to avoid further demonstrations of the famine phenomenon. Covert Bailey is correct: rapid weight loss can make you fatter. The next time I try to reduce my body fat below 2.4 percent, I'll do it very gradually. I won't threaten my body. I'll use gentle persuasion to get my body to give up a little more fat than before.

Bodybuilders striving for maximum muscle with an absolute minimum of fat must learn to deal with the famine phenomenon. The phenomenon becomes more important the closer you come to ultimate muscularity. Take your time in shedding the last remnants of fat for competition. Don't try to lose more than one pound of fat a week. Stick to a balanced diet. Use aerobic exercise. Reduce your calorie consumption *slightly*. Increase your calorie expenditure *slightly*. Your success will depend on how well you deal with the famine phenomenon.

The Sodium Factor

"You weren't as sharp as you were in San Jose," Ralph Countryman told me in Detroit after the 1979 Past-40 Mr. America contest. Earlier in the year I had won my height class, along with the Most Muscular, Best Abdominals and Best Leg awards, at the Past-40 Mr. U.S.A. contest in San Jose, Calif. Ralph is a national and international physique judge, and at that time he was Chairman of

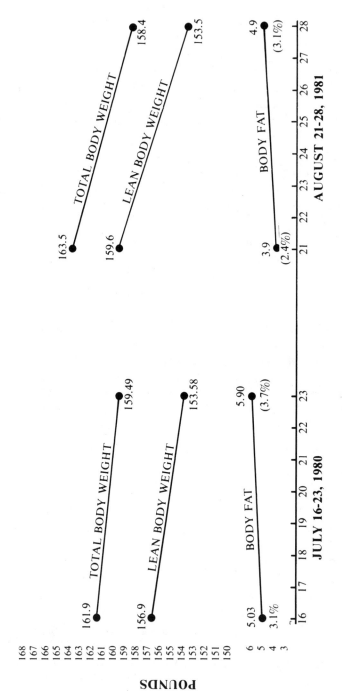

Graph 5. Body composition changes during the weeks of July 16-23, 1980, and August 21-28, 1981. I'm losing weight, but gaining fat.*

*Body composition tests performed by Lovelace Medical Center, Research Division, Albuquerque, New Mexico.

The Famine Phenomenon

the National Physique Judges Committee. So naturally I took his comment seriously. Nevertheless, I was puzzled, because I came to the contest with more muscle than ever before and with my body fat at a rock bottom 2.4 percent.

Several weeks after the contest I received photos taken in Detroit by famous physique photographer Dave Sauer. Ralph was right. My body looked spongy; my definition was blurred. It was as if a film of some kind was covering my body. I saw Dave some months later, after the publication of *Ripped*. He asked me why I hadn't used any of his photos in my book, and then, before I could respond, he answered his own question: "I guess it was because you looked puffy."

Yes, something was definitely wrong in Detroit, but it was more than a year later—at the 1980 Past-40 Mr. America contest in Atlanta, Ga.—that I realized what the problem was. When I got out of bed on the morning of the Atlanta show, the first thing I did was check my condition in the mirror. I thought I was looking a little flat, but I chalked it up to nervousness and poor lighting in the hotel room. There wasn't much I could do about it at that point, anyway, so I tried not to worry.

As I prepared for the Prejudging I still looked a little smooth, but I told myself that it must be my imagination. On the Wednesday before the contest I had had my body composition checked. My body fat was very low and my definition was excellent.

After the Prejudging was completed, however, the first thing my wife, Carol, said to me was, "What happened to your cuts?" Then I knew. The mirrors in the hotel room and in the dressing room were not lying. Something was drastically wrong. But what?

Talking to other bodybuilders later that day further confirmed my fears. Several tactfully told me that they were disappointed. They expected me to be sharper. As I mingled with the crowd and talked to various people, the consensus was that I was puffy and holding water under my skin. This started me thinking. I knew that many bodybuilders restrict fluid intake prior to a contest but, frankly, I hadn't put much stock in the practice. I also knew that consuming excessive salt (sodium chloride) would cause water retention. I hadn't worried about that either, because I never add salt to anything.

I looked back over the last several days. I had been staying at the Atlanta Hilton and had eaten most of my meals at the hotel's excellent salad bar buffet. I thought this was a good idea because I could see exactly what I was getting. For the most part I ate fruit and vegetables. But for breakfast I had poached eggs, just like I do at home. The chef was stationed at the end of the long buffet and cooked the eggs right in front of me. I watched him crack the eggs and drop them into boiling water. I knew I hadn't gotten any salt that way. At home I usually have yogurt with both my noon and evening meals. There was no yogurt on the hotel buffet, but there was plenty of cottage cheese. I thought cottage cheese would be a satisfactory substitute for my usual yogurt and that's what I had for lunch and dinner. On the evening before the contest my wife and I ate in one of the fancy hotel restaurants. I thought I had done all right there, too, because I had broiled fish with a light sauce which seemed harmless enough. So what was the problem?

I discussed the puzzle with my wife. I told her I thought salt might be the problem. We reviewed what I ate before the contest. Carol stopped me when I got to cottage cheese. She told me that cottage cheese is high in sodium. Carol had been more sodium conscious than me. She knew that people with high blood pressure, who must restrict their sodium intake, are advised to limit their consumption of cottage cheese. So that was the answer: cottage cheese.

Of course, once we focused on the sodium factor, it was easy to figure out that some of the vegetables I'd so carefully selected from the hotel buffet were salted. And the delicate sauce on the broiled fish I had the night before the contest also contained salt.

Then it dawned on us what had happened the previous year in Detroit. The night before the contest Carol and I ate at a pleasant little Italian restaurant, where we had eggplant parmigiana. The food was absolutely delicious. I'm sure it was also loaded with salt. I enjoyed it so much that I went back for more the next afternoon before the evening show!

When I got home from Atlanta, I did some research on sodium. I learned that potassium tends to concentrate inside the cells of the body and sodium tends to concentrate in the fluid surrounding the cells. Taking in excess sodium causes an accumulation of sodium outside the cells and pulls water from the cells into the space between the cells. This creates a puffy and bloated appearance. It became clear that seemingly minor and innocent dietary changes the last day or two before a contest can torpedo a whole year of preparation.

142

Further research confirmed the wisdom of never adding salt to anything. The daily requirement for sodium is extremely low. Sodium deficiencies are rare because sodium is present in almost all foods. Doctors have kept patients healthy for years on daily sodium intakes as low as 150 milligrams (150 milligrams is approximately the amount of sodium found in ⅛ teaspoon of salt). Most people consume far more sodium than they need. The average person in America eats between one and two teaspoons of salt (5,000 to 10,000 milligrams) a day. People who eat in fast-food restaurants may consume even more. A McDonald's Big Mac contains 1,510 milligrams of sodium and a Kentucky Fried Chicken dinner with three pieces of chicken has 2,128 milligrams.

Processed and prepared foods usually contain added salt. For example, 3½ ounces of fresh, raw peas contains only two milligrams of sodium, but the same amount of processed, canned peas contains 236 milligrams of sodium.

Of course, I checked the sodium content of cottage cheese. One cup of creamed cottage cheese contains 850 milligrams of sodium. But contrast, one cup of whole milk contains only 120 milligrams of sodium. One cup plain yogurt, my lunch and dinner staple, contains only 105 milligrams of sodium. My switch from yogurt to cottage cheese increased by sodium intake eightfold! Who knows how much extra salt I picked up from the vegetables I selected at the buffet and from the sauce on my broiled fish, or from the eggplant parmigiana in Detroit.

And I learned one more fact, a fact that indicates the powerful influence sodium has on water in the body: one part sodium holds *180 parts water*. Clearly, a little sodium can make a big difference, the difference between a sharp, muscular physique and a puffy, bloated appearance.

Selecting food in a strange setting immediately before a contest is like walking through a mine field. I'll be more careful next time. I won't put anything in my mouth unless I know its sodium content.

Don't blow a year's training like I did. Don't step onstage puffy and bloated. Do your homework on sodium. Stick with unprocessed, natual foods and avoid unfamiliar foods, especially the last few days before a contest.

The Last Few Days

I had expected to be better than ever at the 1980 Past-40 Mr. America contest in Atlanta, and with Joe Weider's help I had scheduled photo sessions in California the following week to capture my condition on film. I was to fly from Atlanta to California on Sunday and be photographed on Monday and Tuesday. I planned to maintain my contest condition until the photos were taken. But you know what Robert Burns said about "the best laid schemes o' mice and men." My cottage cheese encounter in Atlanta threw a monkey wrench into the plan. As it turned out I had two days to go from waterlogged in Atlanta to ripped in California. And that's what happened. I'll tell you how I did it.

The few days before and after my Atlanta debacle taught me that the appearance of your physique can be dramatically altered, for better or worse, from day to day and hour to hour. In the week after Atlanta I was photographed four times: Monday afternoon, Tuesday morning, Tuesday afternoon and the following Saturday. I learned and improved in each session. My new awareness of the "water problem," combined with careful observation and fine tuning, allowed me to steadily increase my definition and bring my physique to a razor-sharp peak for the final photo session.

The main thing I had to do was get rid of the excess water under my skin. I started on Sunday morning. I decided to avoid any food that might have salt added. That was relatively easy, once I understood that there's more to controlling sodium intake than keeping your hands off the salt shaker.

Being away from home and eating in restaurants complicates the problem, because you can't be sure what's salted and what isn't. You have to assume that almost everything served in a restaurant has salt added. To be safe I stuck mainly with eggs, plain baked potatoes and fresh fruit. I was especially careful to stay away from sauces, mixtures of any kind (including omelettes) and, of course, cottage cheese. My rule was: "if you don't know the sodium content, don't eat it."

I made a mental note that when I got home I would buy a book that listed the sodium content of various foods. For the time being, though, I decided that I'd be safe if I ate whole, natural foods with nothing added. That was a good plan. Nature doesn't put excess

144

sodium in food. Modern man does.

Fortunately, I didn't have to worry about calories. My body fat was already quite low. A bodybuilder should get his or her body fat down to a minimum level a week or 10 days before a contest. There are plenty of things to do in the last few days without having to struggle with a low-calorie diet. Since my body fat wasn't a problem, I could consume enough calories to supply my energy needs.

I ate just about all I wanted, but I was careful about my food volume. It wouldn't do to show up for the pictures with my waist sticking out. I ate a normal amount, but I didn't overeat.

The natural foods I ate were not only low in sodium, they had the advantage of fast transit time. Due to the fiber content, this type of food moves through your system rapidly and keeps your bowels open. I was careful not to eat anything that would make me constipated. I wanted to show up for the pictures with my intestinal tract relatively empty and my waist small.

Since I knew that constipation can be a problem when you're traveling and can't move about freely, I also made it a point to stay active. This helped keep my bowels open and my waist small and tight. Good bowel function, of course, would also help me to get rid of excess salt and water.

After a breakfast of two poached eggs, two slices of toast (a mistake—bread contains sodium), grapefruit and coffee, I walked and jogged 3½ miles on the hotel track. It was hot in Atlanta and I worked up a good sweat. That made me feel good, because I knew I was getting rid of the water that had ruined my physique.

On Sunday morning I also began to watch my fluid intake. I didn't stop drinking entirely; I simply didn't do any unnecessary drinking. At this point I didn't know how much I would need to limit my water intake. My physique had been very sharp at home when I was drinking normally. I thought it would be enough to simply watch my fluid intake, stay active and eliminate salt from my diet. As time wore on, however, I decided to restrict my fluid intake a bit more. I learned that your physique is sharper when you're slightly dehydrated.

I had an apple and a glass of wine on the plane, but I didn't eat the meal. Food served on airplanes almost always contains excess sodium. When I got to California I had three over-easy eggs, a baked potato and coffee. After eating I took about a one-hour nap.

When I got up I checked my physique. I could tell I was on the right track. I was looking better. Restricting my sodium intake for only one day made a noticeable difference in my physique. I had two more eggs, a glass of milk and another baked potato before I went to bed.

When I got up on Monday morning I checked my physique again. I still needed to lose more water. For breakfast I had three eggs, two pieces of toast (probably a mistake), one-half cantaloupe and a cup of coffee. I decided against milk and didn't drink any water.

Later that morning I did a light workout at Gold's Gym to help me sweat and lose more water. By chance, I ran into Mike Mentzer at Gold's. I told him I was scheduled for a photo session that afternoon with Joe Weider and I was trying to get rid of subcutaneous water. Mike gave me two good suggestions. He said sunbathing would make me sweat and help me lose the water from under my skin. He also suggested a low-volume, high-carbohydrate meal without water an hour before the photo session. I decided to take Mike's first bit of advice: I laid out in the sun by the Holiday Inn pool for an hour. Unfortunately, the sun wasn't very hot, so I didn't sweat much. I didn't take Mike's suggestion regarding the high-carb meal, however. I was still carrying excess water, and I didn't think extra carbs would be advisable. Later in the week, when the excess water was gone, Mike's suggestion about the carbs came in handy.

My first photo session was under Joe Weider's supervision at Bob Gardner's studio. Frankly, I was disappointed. The lights made me sweat profusely. This told me that I was still carrying too much water under my skin. Joe and Bob Gardner worked hard, but there really wasn't anything they could do. I just wasn't ready. The main thing I got out of that session was some excellent posing tips from Joe Weider. Fortunately, I had more time and more photo sessions coming up. I was determined to be better the next day when Bill Reynolds was scheduled to photograph me on the beach and at Gold's in the morning and in a mountain setting during the afternoon.

To be ready the next day I had to get rid of more water. I didn't want to be disappointed again. In the afternoon, after the session at Bob Gardner's studio, I had a cup of coffee, but I didn't drink anything else. Coffee has a diuretic effect so I wasn't afraid of drinking it. That evening I had a glass of wine (wine also has a diuretic effect) and a lettuce, tomato and egg salad. I had a little of the house dressing on my salad. That was a slip, because I didn't know the sodium content of the salad dressing. I also had a plain baked potato. In addition to the wine, I drank half a glass of milk and half a glass of water. That was it. I had no other fluids.

Later that evening Mike Mentzer dropped by the Holiday Inn and we traded books. I gave him a copy of *Ripped* and he gave me a copy of his *Heavy Duty Journal*. Mike thought his book might help me get ready for the photo sessions the next day. He was right. His section on salt, water and blood volume is excellent. I chuckled when I read that a salty appetizer in Acapulco almost cost Mike his Mr. Universe victory. His experience was much like mine in Atlanta. The salt-laden appetizer blurred Mike's physique to the extent that Frank Zane, who was doing the TV commentary for CBS Sports, ran backstage after Prejudging and asked Mike what he'd done to lose his cuts. Fortunately, Mike's shape, size and symmetry gave him the victory anyway. But like me, he learned a valuable lesson.

In any event, Mike's *Heavy Duty Journal* gave me confidence that I was doing the right things to prepare for the next day. That evening I bundled up in my sweat suit and jogged up and down the stairs of the Holiday Inn four times—28 flights in all. That helped; it made me sweat and kept my bowels functioning. Later that evening I drank two small cups of water. I didn't eat or drink anything else.

The first thing I did when I got up the next morning was to check my physique in the mirror. I was definitely looking better. My skin was thin and tight and my vascularity was good. I thought a little more dehydration would do the job.

I had a nectarine at about 6:30 a.m. and breakfast a little after 7. It consisted of two eggs, a piece of toast, half a cantaloupe and a cup of coffee. I didn't drink water or any other fluids. After breakfast I went for a walk to help digest my breakfast and get rid of a little more water. At 8:30 I met Bill Reynolds at Gold's.

We spent most of the morning taking pictures on the beach and under the skylight at Gold's. I knew I was looking good when I attracted a crowd at Gold's. Many people, including Andreas Cahling, Kent Kuehn and Lou Ferrigno, told me that I was ripped. The folks at Gold's are not easily impressed, so I knew things were definitely looking up. But the best was yet to come.

I continued to watch my fluids at lunch. I had two cups of coffee and some fruit. I didn't eat the lettuce the fruit was served on and I didn't drink any water. After lunch I took a short nap.

When I got up I drove to Weider headquarters in Woodland Hills to meet Bill Reynolds for the last photo session of the day. Bill took me to a nearby mountainous area where he's photographed all the top physique champions. He calls it "Reynold's Rock." It's a spectacular setting of giant boulders with nothing but blue sky in the background.

We had to walk and climb about a quarter of a mile to get to the spot. The climb helped me get rid of the last bit of excess water from under my skin. When we finally got set up, I didn't sweat any more even though it was easily 100^0. I was dried out and ready for the photo session. As a matter of fact, by the time we finished I was feeling weak and shaky. The heat and dehydration got to me. Sometime between the morning photo sessions and the end of that afternoon session on Reynold's Rock, I crossed over the illusive line between absolute peak condition and excessive dehydration. Still, it was damned satisfying standing on Reynold's Rock knowing I was absolutely ripped to the bone.

After that I celebrated—three times! I started out with a pint of cold milk at a 7-Eleven on the way back to the Weider offices. Boy, did that milk taste good! Later that evening, Carol, Matt and I had dinner with Bill and his girlfriend. The part that I remember enjoying the most was drinking the water. The third celebration came on the way back to the Holiday Inn. We stopped off a Zucky's Restaurant, a favorite of the Santa Monica muscle crowd. I quenched my thirst some more and satisfied my sweet tooth at the same time. I had three cups of decaffeinated coffee, a large glass of milk, a delightful piece of cheesecake, a tasty dish of frozen yogurt, and when my son fell asleep, I topped it all off by eating his jello and whipped cream.

There was a surprise waiting for me when I got back to our room. I looked in the mirror and my veins were popping out all over. I was super vascular and cut. At first I thought that was strange in view of the fact I'd just eaten and drank about all I could hold. Then I began to think about Mike Mentzer's suggestion that I have a low-volume, high-carbohydrate meal before my photo session. The water and food, especially the desserts, apparently increased my blood volume and made me more vascular. It probably made my muscles rounder and fuller as well. I wondered if

I would have looked even better on Reynold's Rock if I'd taken Mike's advice.

This thought was still rolling around in my mind when we arrived home in Albuquerque the next day. I talked to Carol about it, and we decided that I should give it a try while I was still in top shape. We contacted a local photographer who agreed to take some shots of me the following weekend. We scouted out a terrific location in the foothills east of Albuquerque. I used the next few days to prepare for the last, and what turned out to be the best, photo session.

In spite of that one afternoon and evening of celebrating, my body fat was still rock bottom. I didn't have to worry about that. I consumed a normal amount of calories. I ate a few more carbohydrates than I did in California because I wanted to be sure the glycogen in my muscles was fully restored. Remember, muscle is 70 percent water. Each gram of carbohydrate stored in your muscles in the form of glycogen holds three grams of water. This makes your muscles full and round. It's important, however, not to let caloric intake get ahead of your energy expenditure. If that happens, the water in your muscles will spill over into the space under your skin and make you look puffy. On the other hand, if you starve yourself before a contest, you'll drain the water out of your muscles. Your muscles won't be round and full; they'll be flat. It's another fine line that you must walk in order to reach peak condition.

When I got home to Albuquerque, my muscles were stiff and sore from the four posing sessions before the cameras in two days. I decided not to work out before the pictures were taken on Saturday. I stayed active by walking and posing. I used my extra time to practice the posing tips Joe Weider gave me.

I didn't train before the last photo session for the same reason I don't train the last few days before a contest. Training uses up the glycogen in the muscles and it takes at least 48 hours for the glycogen to be fully restored. Resting the last few days before a contest gives your final training efforts a chance to have a positive effect. In a manner of speaking, it lets the cream come to the top.

I continually monitored my condition in the mirror. I kept my sodium intake low. I kept myself normally hydrated. I didn't eat or drink anything that would make me waterlogged like I was in Atlanta, so I didn't have the problem of getting rid of excess water. In spite of my celebrating in California, I continued to look sharp as the weekend approached.

I waited until noon on Friday to restrict my fluid intake. I drank a cup of coffee with my dinner and had a small glass of wine later in the evening. I didn't drink anything else. On Saturday morning I got up at 5 a.m., had a cup of coffee, and walked and jogged about two miles to sweat and get my bowels moving.

The major change I made involved my last meal. I followed Mike Mentzer's advice and had a low-volume, high-carbohydrate breakfast at 6:30, about three hours before the photo session. I had a banana, two tablespoons of raisins and one tablespoon of sunflower seeds topped with honey. I also had a piece of toast and a cup of coffee. I had no other fluids. That's all it took to put me in absolutely peak condition for my final and best photo session of the year.

The extra carbs kept my blood sugar up and increased my vascularity without making me puffy. The extra carbs may also have filled out my muscles a little by adding to my glycogen stores. However, this can't take place to any great extent in a period as short as three hours. Eating carbohydrates during the week probably did more to make my muscles rounder and fuller than they were in California. The reason the last meal should be low in volume is, of course, so it won't make your stomach protrude.

Photos have been included to show how I looked in each photo session. I think you'll agree that I look good on the beach, that I look better on Reynold's Rock, and that in Albuquerque on Saturday I look the best of all.

Achieving absolute peak condition for a physique contest is a tricky business. It takes practice. You can't learn how to do it by reading this book. You can only learn how to do it by trying it yourself. Here's a check-list of helpful advice to follow:

1) Ease your body fat down to a rock bottom at least a week before the contest, and then eat enough calories and carbohydrates to sustain yourself going into the contest. This will give you energy and fill out your muscles by completely restoring the glycogen supply. Don't fall victim to the famine phenomenon. Remember, starving yourself before a contest will probably make you fatter.

2) Stop training at least two days before the contest, but stay active to maintain a calorie balance and keep your elimination

processes operating properly. Resting allows your glycogen stores to be replenished and gives your muscles a full, tight look.

3) The last week before the contest, don't eat anything with salt added. Stick with whole, natural food with nothing added.

4) Use suntanning, sweating and fluid restriction to come into the contest in peak condition. But don't overdo it. Don't make yourself sick. And don't get so dehydrated that your muscles become flat.

5) About three hours before the Prejudging, have a low-volume, high-carbohydrate meal without water. This gives your muscles a little extra fullness and brings out your vascularity. It also provides the energy you need to perform well during comparison posing.

A few words about steroids: steroids can help a bodybuilder achieve maximum muscle mass with minimum fat, but they complicate the water balance problem. Steroids, especially the oral type, cause water retention. If you decide to use steroids, I suggest that you cut your dosage way back the last two weeks. And remember one more thing. Any amount of muscle you gain from steroids, you'll probably lose when you stop taking them. And for a time afterwards, your ability to build muscle tissue will be less than it was before you started taking steroids. Long-term, permanent muscle must be built without steroids.

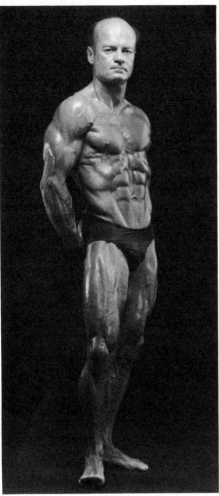

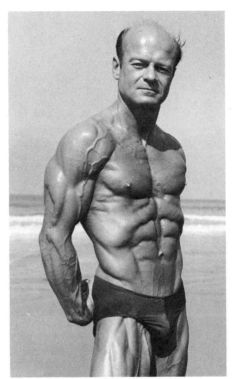

The next morning on the beach I looked better. *Photo by Bill Reynolds.*

Here's how I looked during the first photo session on Monday. Excess water is blurring my definition. *Photo by Bob Gardner.*

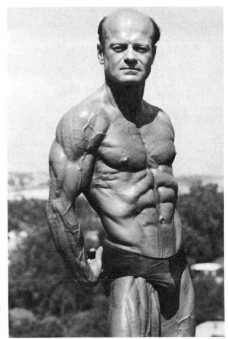

By Tuesday afternoon I'd lost the last bit of excess water from under by skin. On Reynold's Rock I was ripped to the bone. *Photo by Bill Reynolds.*

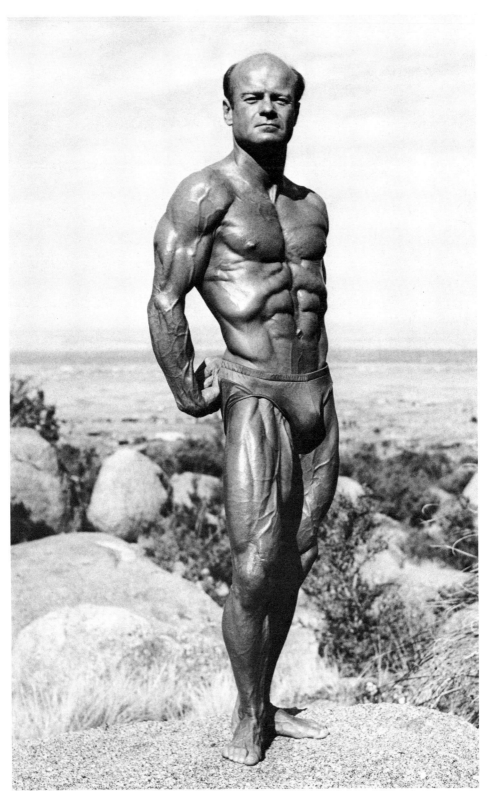

On Saturday in Albuquerque I looked best of all. *Photo by Allen Hughes.*

"Every calling is great, when greatly pursued."
                                    —Oliver Wendell Holmes

"A musician must make music, an artist must paint, a poet must write, if he is to be ultimately happy. What a man can *be, he* must *be."*
                                    —Abraham Maslow

PART FOUR
Training Psychology

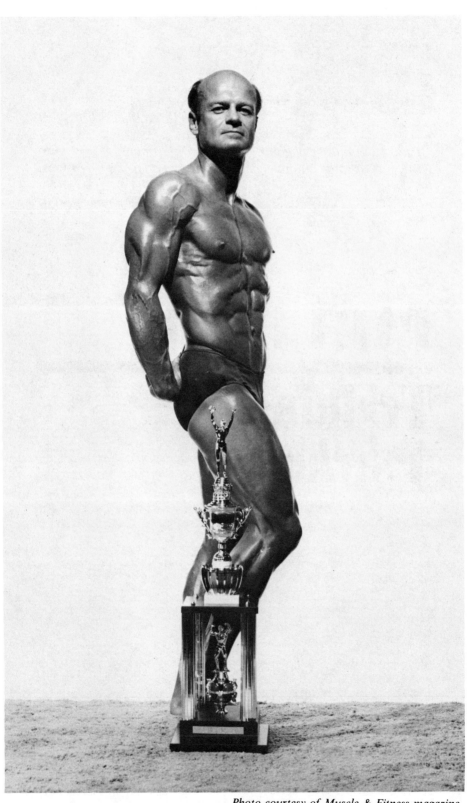

Photo courtesy of Muscle & Fitness magazine.

PART FOUR: TRAINING PSYCHOLOGY

Winning

As George Sheehan says, "We each have a role to play—our own." To the extent we play that role to the best of our ability, we're winners. Despite what some would have us believe, champions are—for the most part—born, not made. Few of us have the genetic potential to be Mr. Olympia or Mr. America, but almost all of us have bodybuilding strong points. For example, no amount of diet and training will give me broad shoulders like Dennis Tinerino's or long biceps like Larry Scott's. On the positive side, however, I inherited the ability to develop good forearms and calves—problem areas for many people—from my father. Most of us have plenty of potential and we can all improve. Our task is to get the most out of ourselves, to be the best bodybuilders we can be.

Not long ago the man who does my photo processing asked me how long it takes to build a body like Arnold's. "You should start before conception," I told him. We both laughed, but it's true. Parents have a lot to do with whether someone can become a bodybuilding champion. Heredity determines your bone structure and the amount of muscle that can be attached to your frame. The digestive system you're born with also determines, to an extent, whether you have a tendency to store fat.

Nevertheless, it does no good to blame your parents for whatever shortcomings they may have bestowed on you. It's a lot more productive to concentrate on your assets. The bottom line is that we're all born with a certain amount of potential—often much more than we realize. The "before" pictures of Bill Pearl, Arnold Schwarzenegger and many other muscle greats show that old-timer Earle E. Liederman was correct when he said, "You never know just how far you can go once your hands touch a barbell."

It's almost axiomatic that after every physique contest there will be at least five competitors who think they were shafted by the judge. Each feels he or she should have won. Each blames the judges for what went wrong. Don't misunderstand, judges are human; they make mistakes. Still, their job is to pick a winner, and they do the best job they can.

Second-guessing the judges rarely helps. It's better to assess your performance objectively to determine whether you improved on previous efforts and to look for ways to do better next time.

I've been attending the Mr. America contest since 1953. Only one person can win, but as I see it, there really are no losers. Every bodybuilder good enough to stand in the Mr. America lineup is a winner. Nevertheless, every year I see top-flight bodybuilders going away from the Mr. America contest feeling like losers. I understand their disappointment, but I wish they could see their performance in a more positive light. Only one man takes the Mr. America crown home, but many more go away winners. It may be that the real winner, the guy who really benefits from the contest, is the happy 10th-place finisher who knows he did his best, better than ever before, and takes joy in the prospect of doing even better next time.

George Sheehan believes that "competition is simply each of us seeking our absolute best with the help of each other." As he sees it, the purpose of competition isn't to beat someone else, but to get the best out of ourselves. Good competition makes a person work harder. This is the philosophy of Kathy Tuite, a world-class competitor in both powerlifting and bodybuilding. She says, "You can't let losing bother you much. Competition goads me into really pushing myself through those extra reps or sprinting up a few more hills."

I know it isn't easy to look at competition this way, especially if you have a chance to win the top prize. Bill Rodgers, in all honesty, probably doesn't wish Alberto Salazar well in the Boston Marathon, and I'd be surprised if Chris Dickerson and Tom Platz were pulling for Franco Columbu to do well at the 1981 Mr. Olympia. Be that as it may, we'd have more "winners" if more bodybuilders competed not to beat someone else, but to get the best out of themselves. Ask yourself this question: is the main purpose of a bodybuilding contest to pick a winner or is it to help all the competitors be the best they can be?

I've learned that you have to look beyond the judges' score sheets to separate the real winners from the losers. At a state contest I judged recently, a woman competitor came up to me afterwards and asked, "What's wrong with my physique?" I told her truthfully that I thought she looked good. Before I could add anything further she wheeled around and stomped away. She placed high, but obviously she thought she should have placed higher.

Backstage later I was shocked to find blood all over the place. Upset by the decision, her boyfriend had rammed his fist through a window. He apparently severed an artery, because his blood was splattered all along the hallway leading to the exit. It was a gory mess. I headed for the parking lot shaking my head in dismay.

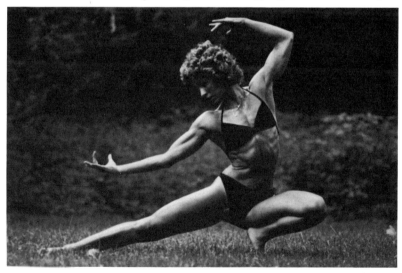

Kathy Tuite uses competition to get the best out of herself.
Photo by John Underwood.

At a recent contest I judged in the East, the Past-40 Mr. USA, I talked to another competitor who had lost. This fellow placed second in his weight class. Yet he was all smiles—and for good reason. I'd seen him compete about a year earlier. This time he had more muscle and a new posing routine which really turned the audience on. He'd been working hard, and it showed. He radiated enthusiasm as he told me that he was now planning to compete in the Past-40 Mr. America contest later in the year. He didn't mind placing second, because he knew he was better than ever before, and he was anxious to make further improvement for the Past-40 Mr. America. In my book this competitor was a winner, even though he hadn't finished first.

"Personal effort is the most important thing," Japan's premier marathoner, Toshihiko Seko, said in an interview with *Running* magazine. "You must run for yourself. I'm striving to reach my full potential, not necessarily to win or set world records." In running and bodybuilding, that's a winning philosophy. Strive to be the best you can be, and you'll be a winner. Remember, your most important competitor is you.

Why I Train

Sure, I train for the usual reasons—to look better, feel better, live longer—but there's more to it than that. The reasons why I train have evolved over the years. They're different now than they were when I started training in my teens.

George Sheehan says that health and fitness doesn't motivate people, that people won't exercise just because it's good for them. Come to think of it, if health alone was enough, more people would probably be training. Something else does seem to be required. Sheehan says it's inspiration.

When I started training at 12 or 13, my motivation was to be stronger than my school buddies. I was small for my age and I think I felt a little inferior. I see the same thing in my son when he plays with the big kid across the street. The other day he called me at the office and asked me to give him a workout program so he could "get some muscle." I might fantasize that he wants to follow in my footsteps, but I know what he really wants is the approval of his peers. The bigger and stronger kids *inspire* him to want "some muscle."

By the time I was a sophomore in high school I was stronger than the guys I ran around with, so I raised my sights. I will never forget a high school awards assembly in which an upper classman was honored for winning the State High School Pentathlon Championship, a five-event contest consisting of push-ups, chin-ups, jump reach, bar vault and 300-yard shuttle run. Seeing that boy get his award as the whole school applauded inspired me. I made up my mind that I'd win that award the next year—and I did.

In later years, lifting champions like Norbert Schemansky, Tommy Kono, Dave Sheppard, Isaac Berger and Chuck Vinci inspired me. Now, bodybuilding champions like Frank Zane, Mike Mentzer and Boyer Coe inspire me. As I get older I'm motivated by the fact that many of the top champions—Bill Pearl, Ed Corney and Albert Beckles, the World Professional Champion titleholder—are older than I am and still in top shape. Nevertheless, the inspiration I receive from these men isn't the only thing, probably not even the main thing, that keeps me training.

I've been at it so long that training is part of me; a psychologist would probably say it's become part of my ego structure. Taking my weight training away would be like cutting off my arm or taking away a key component of my personality. My bodybuilding is an important part of the positive view I have of myself. It's part of what allows me to say, "I'm OK."

A recent conversation with an old training partner reminded me that lifting becomes an important part of one's self-image. My friend and I lost track of one another after we stopped training together 10-12 years ago. When we met again, we chatted all afternoon to catch up on the goings-on in each other's life. He has never stopped training. He's been working out in his home gym since he stopped training in my garage. It was fascinating to hear him explain why he still trains. He expressed many of the same things I felt about my training.

My friend is married to a nurse, and they have a 12-year-old daughter who is a champion gymnast. His teaching career has gone quite well; he's in line for a principalship. He's 38 years old (and I was envious to see he still has a full head of hair). He's broad-shouldered and handsome. Everything is going his way and, one assumes, will continue to whether or not he trains.

Working out is an integrating factor in my friend's life. He says it's like a ball of string that winds its way through his life, tying everything together. He feels like everything is all right as long as he's still lifting weights. He sees himself as a lifter. When he stands before a group of students, parents or teachers, it's important to him that he looks good. He realizes that the people in the audience don't think much about it, but it's still important to him. He likes the feeling of being strong, of having big muscles and a flat stomach. He wouldn't feel right facing the world with atrophied muscles and a pot belly.

I know how he feels, because I feel the same way. Most of the people I come in contact with don't know, and don't care, that I'm a bodybuilder. It makes little difference to them whether my body fat is three percent or 30 percent. It does make a difference to me, however, and that's what counts.

My friend also likes the feeling of control he gets from training. When he's in his garage working out, he's in charge. Boxer Sugar Ray Leonard expressed the same thought recently in *Sports Illustrated:* "a lot of time, out of training, I don't even know where I am. Training gives me sanity. That's the one time in my life when I know what I'm doing."

Sugar Ray and my friend have a point. So many things these days are beyond our control. That's why it's important to have a sanctuary where we're in control, even if it's only in the gym. The hour or so I spend in my gym calms me for the rest of my day. Controlling the stress that I undergo in my gym fortifies me for the chaos on the outside.

And my friend and I agree on another thing: we're both going to end up with gigantic balls of string. "I'm not sure what I'm going to do with mine," my friend said, smiling.

Success Is What Keeps You Training

What has kept me training for more than 30 years? As I said earlier, I've trained for so long that it's part of me. I'd be lost if I didn't train. Yet, as I look back, I see things that got my training off on the right foot and kept me at it year after year.

Probably the number one factor in training longevity, in staying with your training, is setting and achieving realistic goals. The strength of one's motivation depends, for the most part, on past success. A person usually won't aspire to success as a bodybuilder,

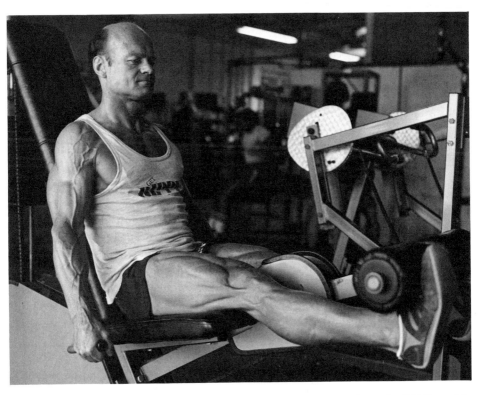

The time I spend in the gym calms me for the rest of my day. *Photos by Bill Reynolds.*

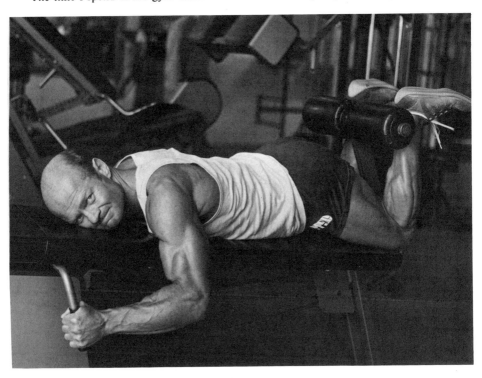

or anything else, unless he or she has already had some success along the way. In general, people set their goals a little higher than they think they can go, and that's OK. Others, however, aim well below their capacity to achieve, or they set their goals unrealistically high. These are the bodybuilders who drop out.

Almost everyone makes good gains when he or she first starts bodybuilding. So most people have that all-important initial success. Where the beginning bodybuilder aims next determines, in large part, whether training motivation continues.

At the 1979 Mr. Olympia contest in Columbus, Ohio, I sat next to a young man who was literally bubbling over with enthusiasm. As he marveled at the likes of Frank Zane, Mike Mentzer, Boyer Coe and the other marvelous physiques onstage, he told me that he couldn't wait to get back to the gym, because he was going to be Mr. America, Mr. Universe and Mr. Olympia. I don't know what happened to him, but it's my guess that unless he lowered his sights, at least initially, he's now an ex-bodybuilder.

It's fine to know, in the back of your mind, that you'd like to be Mr. Olympia, but you must remember that the longest journey begins with the first step. That young bodybuilder should have aimed at a novice contest. If he was successful against other beginners, he then could have raised his sights to the next level. In that way he'd establish a pattern of success that would take him as far as his potential would allow.

Fortunately, my training efforts have been continually rewarded. Like other beginners, my body responded to my initial efforts with the weights. After I achieved my first goal—to be as strong as my friends—I trained for, and won, the State High School Pentathlon Championship I mentioned earlier. That was a big win for me. I did more push-ups and chin-ups than any other boy in the state. On the jump reach I went higher than anybody else as well. The fourth event was the bar vault; you pull-up and flip your body over a high bar. I bar vaulted as high as I could reach on my tip toes. The only event I didn't do well in was the 300-yard shuttle run, and that didn't bother me too much because I wasn't really interested in running and hadn't worked at it.

Looking back, I realize that training for and winning the State High School Pentathlon established a pattern for me to follow the rest of my life. That victory taught me how tremendously satisfying it is to set a goal, work hard, and then succeed. The local newspaper ran a story headlined, "Bass is Strongest." I was on my way.

My next goal was to the win the city weightlifting championship. I was successful there, too, but at that point I almost bit off more than I could chew. I began to set unrealistic goals for myself. I remember telling a friend that I'd be disappointed if I didn't become a world champion.

About that time I went to an Olympic lifting contest in El Paso, Texas with the 1955 Mr. America, Steve Klisanin. At that contest I became one of the youngest lifters in the country to clean and jerk 300 pounds. That set my hopes soaring. I must have been popping off about the great things I was going to do, because I remember that Klisanin brought me abruptly back the earth. He said, "You're no Norbert Schemansky." (Schemansky was then US and World Champion.) Taken aback, I asked Klisanin how he knew. I don't remember his answer, but as it turned out, he was right.

I think Steve was trying to tell me that I should focus on state and regional championships, and be successful there before I started thinking about higher level competition. That's what I eventually did. I became New Mexico champion, Southwest champion, Rocky Mountain champion and placed second in the Teenage National Championships and the Jr. National Championships. As a young lifter, if I'd refused to take the cue from Klisanin, and instead set my cap on becoming another Norbert Schemansky or else, I probably would have become discouraged and given up long ago.

How successful you are on a workout-to-workout basis is also important. You should try to make every training session a satisfying and rewarding experience. Structure your workouts so they produce a feeling of accomplishment. An important part of each workout should be the setting of realistic and attainable goals for the next workout.

After every training session I write my goals for the next session in my training diary. I don't put down anything complicated. While the workout is fresh in my mind, I simply use an arrow to indicate whether I should repeat a movement with the same weight and reps, or add weight and reps, or whatever. Furthermore, I don't hesitate to lower the weight or reps when I get ahead of myself. This procedure helps assure a positive experience next time.

I try to move from one training success to another. Remember, the strength of your training motivation depends on your past success. If your workouts are filled with failure, you'll eventually get

165

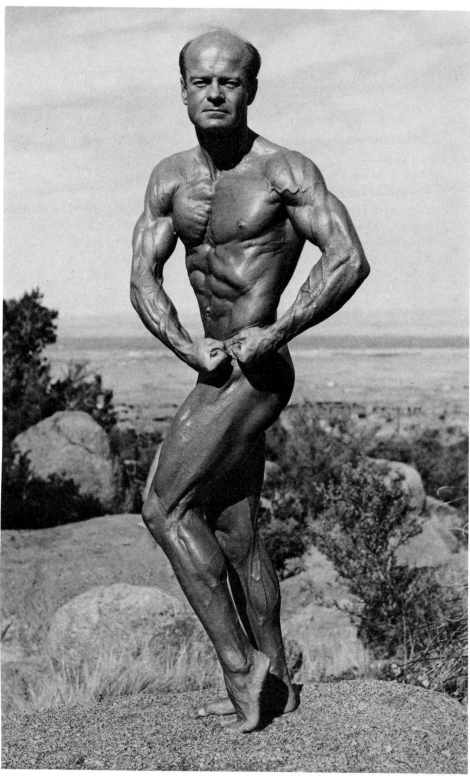

The strength of one's motivation depends, for the most part, on past success. Fortunately, my training efforts have been continually rewarded. *Photo by Allen Hughes.*

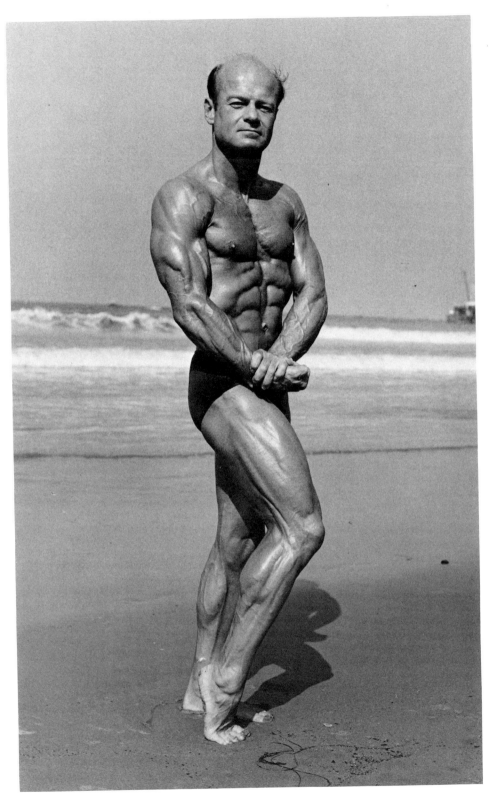

It's tremendously satisfying to set a goal, work hard, and then succeed. *Photo by Bill Reynolds.*

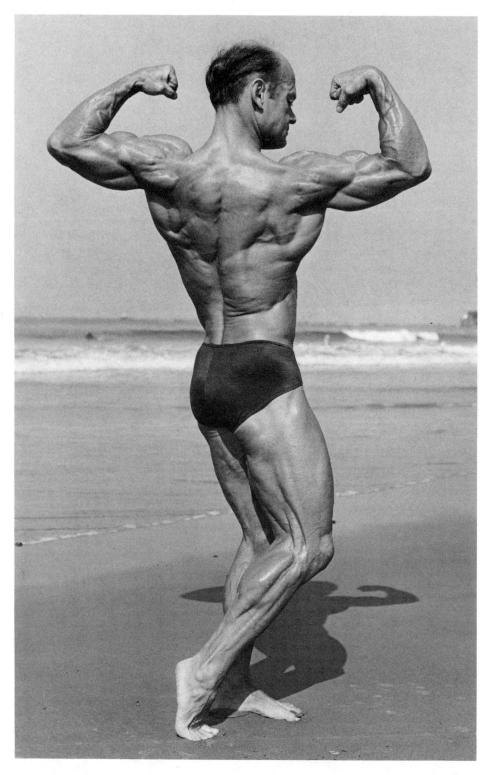

Set reasonable goals; that's the key. *Photo by Bill Reynolds.*

disgusted and quit. On the other hand, if you continually achieve your training goals, you reinforce the training habit, and you keep training year after year. Set reasonable goals; that's the key.

Most of us are creatures of habit. Our day-to-day activities are largely routine. We tend to develop an orderly pattern of living which leads to the development of habits that become an established part of our lifestyle. In bodybuilding, if you get off to a good start and build on your successes in a realistic way, like I did, your training eventually becomes a habit, like brushing your teeth. Bodybuilding becomes a rewarding part of your life, a part you don't want to give up.

There's another factor that keeps you training, and it may be the most important factor of all. You must enjoy training. If you don't enjoy it, you probably won't continue.

In a recent article in *The Runner* magazine, Frank Shorter wrote that from January 1970 to December 1980, he averaged 120 miles of running a week. That's 17 miles a day for more than a decade! Shorter gave a number of reasons why he put so much time and effort into his training, but he ended by saying he couldn't have done it if he simply didn't like to run. "In fact," Shorter wrote, "I suspect sometimes that my long-term goals may simply be excuses to be able to run more than I might otherwise." It's a lot easier to keep bodybuilding if you enjoy the physical act of lifting weights.

I like to train. I like stretching my limits a little each workout, lifting a little more than the time before. I like being completely absorbed in a workout. I like the feeling of mastery over my body that training gives me. I like feeling my muscles contract. I like the full feeling of blood in my muscles and the warm, used feeling that comes after a hard set. And I like the tired, satisfied feeling that comes after the workout is over.

My workouts are a means to an end, but they're an end as well. I like being in peak condition, but I also like the process of getting there. Some workouts are more enjoyable than others, but they're all important to me. Because as George Sheehan has written, "Happiness, we come to discover, is found in the pursuit of happiness."

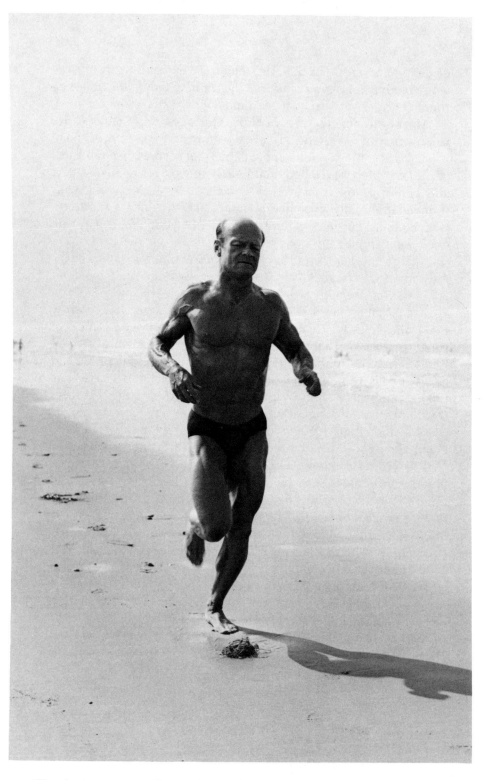

"Happiness we come to discover is found in the pursuit of happiness." George Sheehan
Photo by Bill Reynolds.

OTHER BOOKS BY CLARENCE BASS

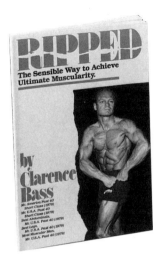 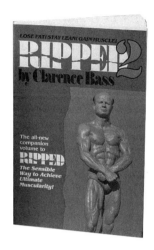 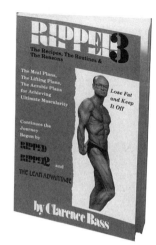

THE RIPPED SERIES

Clarence Bass' quest for lifelong leanness begins with the *Ripped series.* Your journey should begin there as well.

In *Ripped*, Clarence explains, step-by-step, how he reduced his body fat to 2.4% and won his class in the Past-40 Mr. America contest. This is the basic diet book for bodybuilders and fitness-minded individuals.

Ripped 2 explains staying lean, aerobics, building muscle, peaking and bodybuilding psychology. Many say it's the best book ever written on weight training.

Ripped 3 contains detailed comments on 22 meal plans that will make and keep you lean. Plus, it's the break-through book on periodization training for bodybuilders.

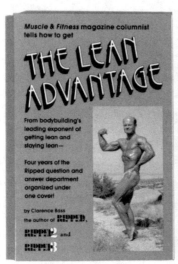

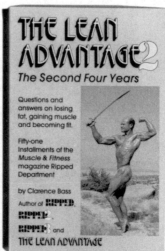

THE LEAN ADVANTAGE SERIES

Do you have questions about losing fat, getting fit, healthy lifestyle, aging or anything relating to diet and exercise?

Chances are the answers are in The Lean Advantage series, where 155 installments of Clarence Bass'

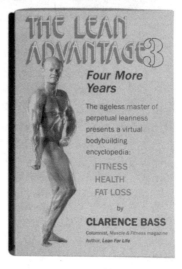

popular question and answer column, The Ripped Department, are collected. Taken together, the three books (The Lean Advantage 1, 2 & 3) constitute an virtual encyclopedia of the bodybuilding and fitness lifestyle.

Here are some of the topics covered: bodyfat tests, successful dieting, muscle building, aerobics, exercise physiology, motivation, preventable diseases, aging and much, much more,

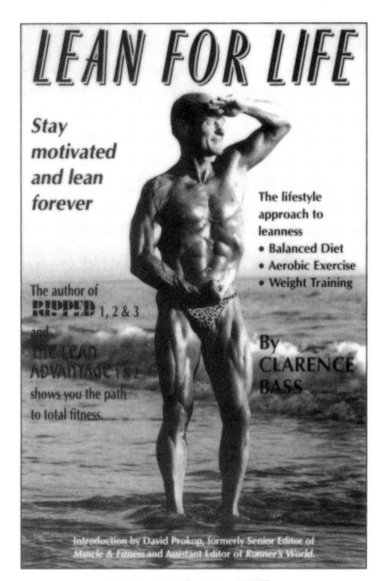

The lifestyle approach to leanness
- Balanced Diet
- Aerobic Exercise
- Weight Training

By CLARENCE BASS

The author of **RIPPED** 1, 2 & 3 and THE LEAN ADVANTAGE 1 & 2 shows you the path to total fitness.

Introduction by David Prokop, formerly Senior Editor of Muscle & Fitness and Assistant Editor of Runner's World.

LEAN FOR LIFE

The fitness trend is toward balanced training—strength and endurance. Clarence Bass leads the way with *LEAN FOR LIFE*. He explains, day-by-day, how to combine weights and aerobics to achieve total fitness. What's more, he shows how to stay motivated—and lean—forever. He presents a lifestyle approach that *will make you lean for life*.

Don't miss a single step on the road to permanent leanness. Read all of Clarence Bass' books.

Turn the page for more information and where to order

Clarence Bass'

RIPPED™ Enterprises

We are your source for bodybuilding, fitness, health, motivation, diet and fat loss information

Please visit us on the Internet at http://www.cbass.com.

You'll find not only information about our books and other products, but also more about Clarence Bass' background and training career, his diet and training philosophy in brief, frequently asked questions, late news — and new articles by Clarence Bass (a new article at the beginning of each month).

Ripped Enterprises
528 Chama N.E.
Albuquerque, NM 87108 USA
Phone: 505-266-5858
Fax: 505-266-9123

Also available from
Clarence Bass' RIPPED Enterprises

❖ Posing Trunks

❖ Women's
   Posing Suits

❖ Audio tapes

❖ Videos and DVDs

❖ Color Photos

❖ Food
   Supplements

❖ Selected
   Books

❖ Personal
   Consultations

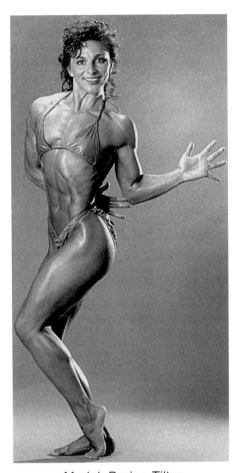

Model: Dorine Tilton

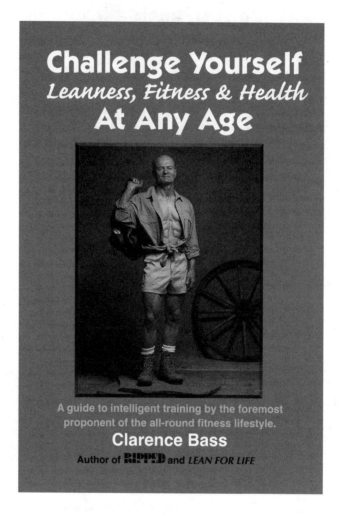

Challenge Yourself
Leanness, Fitness & Health
At Any Age

A guide to intelligent training by the foremost
proponent of the all-round fitness lifestyle.

Clarence Bass

Author of **RIPPED** and *LEAN FOR LIFE*

Challenge Yourself is Clarence Bass' latest book. The key to becoming—and staying— lean, fit and healthy is to continually challenge yourself in an intelligent and thoughtful way. That's what this book is about. It explains how Clarence has continued to improve for more than 45 years—and how you can follow suit. The other books get you started and this book will keep you going.

Cutting edge, ***Challenge Yourself*** includes psychologically sound techniques for staying motivated, the latest developments in diet and nutrition, detailed new routines for beginners and intermediates (weights only), Clarence's current routine, athlete-type strength training, high-intensity aerobics, longevity and health topics, and exciting personal profiles.